a LOVED ONE *Has* DEMENTIA

---

*A Comforting Companion
for Family and Friends*

EVELINE HELMINK

Translated by Laura Vroomen

THE EXPERIMENT
NEW YORK

Library of Congress Cataloging-in-Publication Data

Names: Helmink, Eveline, author. | Vroomen, Laura, translator.
Title: When a loved one has dementia : a comforting companion for family and friends / Eveline Helmink ; translation by Laura Vroomen.
Other titles: Niet vergeten. English
Description: New York : The Experiment, 2023. | "Originally published as Niet vergeten in the Netherlands by Kosmos Uitgevers. First published in North America in revised form by The Experiment, LLC, in 2023"--copyright page. | Includes bibliographical references.
Identifiers: LCCN 2023016020 (print) | LCCN 2023016021 (ebook) | ISBN 9781615199341 (hardcover) | ISBN 9781615199358 (ebook)
Subjects: LCSH: Dementia--Popular works. | Dementia--Patients--Family relationships--Popular works.
Classification: LCC RC521 .H4513 2023 (print) | LCC RC521 (ebook) | DDC 616.8/31--dc23/eng/20230504
LC record available at https://lccn.loc.gov/2023016020
LC ebook record available at https://lccn.loc.gov/2023016021

ISBN 978-1-61519-934-1
Ebook ISBN 978-1-61519-935-8

Jacket and text design by Jack Dunnington
Author photograph by Dana van Leeuwen
Translation by Laura Vroomen

Manufactured in the United States of America

First printing August 2023
10 9 8 7 6 5 4 3 2 1

*So many were gone. In the end, everybody had left
and no one danced with no one in the light of the setting sun.*

—Toon Tellegen

CONTENTS

INTRODUCTION

A few things I'd like to say first

Above my desk hangs a photo of my mother as a young woman. She smiles at my father, who's behind the camera. The sea wind blows her long, deep-brown hair across her face, obscuring her lively, dark eyes. Her mouth is slightly open, as if she's saying something—something sweet. They're on the island of Ameland on what must have been a day in early spring: My mother has wrapped my father's striped scarf around her neck. Of all the photos and slides that my father took of her during their years together—and there are *many*—this is my favorite image. She looks so carefree there on the beach, the place she loves the most. She looks beautiful to me. She feels very close. I often gaze at this portrait when the morning light falls on it or when, in the early hours, the burning candles on my desk cast a flickering glow on the wall. As my fingers hover over my keyboard, I imagine her whispering to me through time: Go on then, write . . .

Her memories are fading and so are mine. When I think of my mother these days, I picture her as a frail little bird without language. Trying to make sense of her words and sentences has become the new normal. I can't remember the exact sound of her voice. Her dark eyes are unfathomable and often drift far beyond the horizon to places I can't see. They look by turns stunned, loving, angry, and sometimes full of tears, sprung from a well deeper and saltier than the sea she can no longer name. My mother—the powerful woman from my childhood, with her outspoken opinions and knowing glances, mischievous smile and swirly handwriting—is lost in time. The further forward we go together, the more memories disappear. The same goes for our memories of her, as well as memories of the two of us. The woman she was fades like a Polaroid developing in reverse.

You may have a loved one with dementia, too. Like me, you've come face-to-face with this illness and everything it sets in motion. You know that talking about dementia involves a lot of stuttering, stammering, and searching for the right thing to say. I don't know if I'll ever find the words to accurately describe what it's like to live with this diagnosis. By writing this book, I'm stepping out onto a tightrope, performing a balancing act between the raw reality of dementia on the one hand and calm, comforting vistas on the other. I feel compelled to write not because I'm an expert but because I want to find a place for dementia in my life: for every single facet of it, candidly, openly, and not buried under fear, sorrow, and powerlessness. I'm convinced that everything you pull out of the shadows and into the light will make life a little lighter, too. And more light is always welcome.

There are plenty of informative books that explain what dementia is and how we can support and care for somebody living with the condition. There are literary books, poignant movies, and websites full of advice. While those resources have been invaluable to me, they don't always offer *solace*. With this book, I hope to bring something new to how we interpret dementia—I'm targeting neither patients nor caregivers, but you: you who also loves someone with dementia, you the family member, partner, friend, or beholder. We're in the same boat. I'd like to add comfort, courage, and resilience to everything you've discovered so far in your encounter with dementia. We share something fundamental, you and I. I hope that you feel seen.

It's been said that when you've met one person with dementia you've met only one person with dementia. It's worth highlighting, because ultimately our stories are each unique, and each person's life is one of a kind. My narrative may not reflect your experiences blow by blow, and perhaps you won't relate to every single detail. But if there's one thing I've learned through the journey, it's this: When all's said and done, we can find universal comfort and recognition in our shared tears. While we may not experience the dementia of our loved ones in the exact same way, I'm not the first and you won't be the last to be impacted by this illness. However deep our feelings of loneliness may be on this journey, I draw solace from the realization that I follow in the footsteps of others who have walked this road before me. We find signs of life along the way. Have you ever been to a lakeshore or a mountaintop and come across a small tower of pebbles, built by human hands? Whenever I happen upon a stack, I feel a connection with a total stranger. Perhaps this book can be such a rock sculpture for you. At the end of the day, all that separates us from one another is time and place.

I'll *never* not be sad that my mother can't be a lucid and engaged part of my life until her very last breath. Although she's still with us, I miss who my mother used to be at the important moments. But equally, I'll never *not* be thankful to her for teaching me, even in the middle of dementia, what really matters: lessons on love and grief, on living with adversity and opportunities, on feeling, becoming, being. It's strange but true that even in pain and sadness, we grow. Even with dementia in our lives, it's possible to enjoy purpose, inner peace, and happiness. That alone is a comfort to me. In an age when we're obsessed with hiding, suppressing, and despising anything that vaguely reminds us of mortality, you'd almost forget.

Not getting mired in sadness, disappointment, and fear can be a challenge. Seeing all sides of dementia, overcoming our resistance and antagonism, and approaching it with curiosity demands an open mind. It's a process of trial and error. You'll cut yourself on sharp edges and stumble over falling rocks, as dementia can be an inhospitable place. But every now and then you'll be able to lean back, turn your face to the sun, and enjoy the view. Perhaps that feels unlikely right now, but you will. You can't choose your battles, but you have more of a choice than you think in how you fight them.

I believe there's more to dementia than the long, dark, endless tunnel that we collectively fear, and I'd like to tell that story. Dementia's one-sided image as sad and gray is as regrettable as it is harmful for both patient and beholder. Anyone confronted with the condition will realize how painful it is, but they also deserve to know that there are glimmers of hope. A person with dementia is more than just the disease—they are a human being and someone who matters. If we can agree on that, we've already come a long way. Nothing we can say or do can take away the dementia. The reality of this illness is that it cares little about our desires, expletives, or tears, but we can certainly make life with dementia a little easier. There will be moments of comfort and connection, humor, levity, and respite. Trust me. You'll be able to draw on unimaginable reserves of strength and resilience, courage and love. During a process that's demanding enough as it is, it's important to focus on these rays of light. They make all the difference when confronted with the dark.

It's not your job or responsibility to discover light or meaning in dementia. This disease doesn't enter your life as a potential lesson, but when it does rear its head, it can teach you a lot. I hope you'll see this book as an invitation, as a helping hand. It's up to you and you alone to decide whether you have the courage or the energy to read. If you're not up for it, I understand. Feel free to give in to your resistance and slam the book shut, and we'll sit side by side in silence for a while. Sometimes that's enough, don't you think?

What it comes down to for me is that I want you to know that you're not forgotten.

One final thing I'd like to say: The story of my mother's dementia, which is woven through this book, isn't mine alone. My father and brothers gave me their generous consent and unconditional trust to write about this emotional subject from my personal perspective, and for that I'm grateful. My father and I see my mother's approval reflected in everything she considered worthwhile.

KNOW YOURSELF

Dementia entered my life by the back door. I don't even know when I first uttered the word "dementia" in relation to my mother and our family. I can't remember when I became fully conscious that it was no longer just an abstract notion, a thing of which I'm aware but have no direct experience. The neurons in my mother's brain had triggered an irreversible process right under our noses, and the illness now manifested as something palpable, concrete, and inexorable. No longer "just another word," dementia became a very present reality. It arrived slowly, imperceptibly, and quietly until suddenly it was simply there.

My mother has dementia.

Perhaps the dementia was already there more than ten years ago when, moments before boarding a flight to Australia, she didn't just hold the boarding passes for a second, like my father asked, but packed them away in an unlikely place in their luggage. My dad was puzzled by that. Perhaps the dementia was already present in the delivery room when I gave birth to my eldest son, who's now in high school, and she held the camera upside down and had no idea which button to press. Perhaps she hadn't been reading a word of any of the books in the big stack beside her chair for ages, and maybe it explains why she kept asking me if I wanted coffee even though I've never liked it in all my forty years. It's all become such a blur that none of us, neither my father, brothers, nor myself, can pinpoint when it started. "How long?" people sometimes ask. We don't know. There are times when that makes me sad; I have no idea, for example, when we had our last *real* conversation, with both of us equally aware of what we said. I can't remember when she last told me "I love you" before her magnificent brain surrendered its first wisp of clarity to the wind.

There's no precise timeline of my mother's illness, no "This is when she got dementia, then we did this or that, and now we're here." At best, we can work our way back and speculate as to when it started. It's only now, many years later, when my mother is no longer living at home, that I can look back and see the mountain we've climbed and the path we've gone down. As we get closer to the valley below, we have a much clearer sense of the endless stream of people who've gone before us. All the shock, dismay, and ignorance, all the sadness, powerlessness, and love—we were certainly not the first to experience these emotions. We weren't alone, no matter how lonely my mother's illness often made us feel.

I realize now it's not unusual that we remained in the dark for so long. There are several reasons, which this book will address, but first among them is this: To those not affected by it, dementia is terra incognita, or unknown territory. It's something for later, something that happens to other people, something you don't want to reflect on too much unless you really have to. Besides, it's a complex condition riddled with false assumptions. Many are unaware that dementia, like cancer, is caused by a defect in the body; it's not a mental disorder, but a physical disease of the brain. "Dementia" is an umbrella term that covers a broad range of symptoms that vary from person to person and change as the illness progresses.

There's no list to check off, no fixed timeline to follow. All we can say with any certainty is that for someone with dementia, time is the greatest enemy. Dementia is a chronic, terminal illness, and a person with dementia will never get better. It is both short- and long-term memory decline, while various other brain functions that we depend on to navigate life break down and ultimately fail altogether. It impacts the patient's life in many areas, from carrying out simple, everyday tasks and having a sense of time and place to understanding the complexity of "normal" social interaction. Eventually, the brain is so badly damaged that the body no longer functions.

The most common form of dementia is Alzheimer's disease. That's why the US organization that strives to "end Alzheimer's and all other dementia" is known simply as the Alzheimer's Association. Dementia is the collective name for dozens of disorders that slowly erode the brain. Maybe your loved one has vascular dementia, Lewy body dementia, frontotemporal dementia, or primary progressive aphasia. In my mother's case, it's still not entirely clear which of the latter two is the culprit. It often takes an autopsy of the brain to arrive at an accurate diagnosis. In the early stages of the illness, even physicians are frequently at a loss. My mother's confusion was initially attributed to her thyroid, to stress, to all kinds of things. And on top of everything else, the symptoms can vary from person to person.

Each human being is unique, with or without dementia. There's no such thing as a typical "demented person" or someone who's "dementing"—terms that are obsolete and no longer fit for purpose, yet still widely used. You live with dementia, but you cannot be reduced to it. I won't go into the many different forms of dementia and their associated symptoms; I don't have the medical expertise or experience to do justice to all the ins and outs. For the simplicity, in this book I'll use the umbrella term "dementia."

According to the World Health Organization (WHO), around fifty million people worldwide are currently living with a form of dementia, and there are some ten million new cases annually. Most people who get dementia are sixty and over, and together, they make up 5 to 8 percent of the global population. There are close to six million people with dementia in the United States, including two hundred thousand who are younger than sixty-five. Those are abstract figures until you stop to think about just how many people they represent, and how many more people care for or worry about a person living with dementia. Tens of millions of individuals with dementia means hundreds of millions of loved ones and beholders both near and far. How come dementia felt so remote until my mother was diagnosed with it?

Dementia has been dubbed "the silent epidemic" because, in reality, it's never far away, only hidden from view. Together, people with dementia and those who love them form a large, invisible web connected by one of the major endemic illnesses of our age. Around the time my first book came out, I began to tentatively talk about my mother's condition in public. Although it wasn't the focus of *The Handbook for Bad Days*, the sadness, powerlessness, and uncertainty over my mother's declining health and my search for comfort, courage, and resilience were already making themselves known in my work. Nearly every time I broached the subject of dementia, I encountered relief and recognition. After a reading there'd always be someone waiting to share their own story or sending me an emotional message on social media or a personal email. Without fail, they would mention how my experience is "recognizable."

It may not be immediately apparent, but right now, there is likely someone in your social circle who's dealing with or knows someone who is suffering from dementia. I know so many people who have, or had, a loved one with dementia. The invisible web has been revealed, liberating me to open up dementia for discussion. I feel a deep connection with them and with you.

For a long time, my mother's incipient dementia was hard to pin down and impossible to talk about. I'll describe the whole process and what it has been like for us later in the book, but at this point, I want to address a broader issue: Why does dementia feel so distant to so many people when it's unfolding right before our eyes? The answer is as simple as it is sobering: because we don't *want* to know.

All of this is tied up in the fear surrounding a dementia diagnosis. It's one of very few conditions in which the first thing we notice is how the thinking mind begins to falter, malfunction, and break down. In most serious illnesses, it's the other way around: the body deteriorates first, while the patient often remains who we've always known and loved right up to the end. Although dementia is also a physical disease, as I mentioned earlier, it's perceived and experienced differently. In many cases, the body will soldier on and facilitate life for some time, while the person we know and love so much—their character, their independence—is leaving us bit by bit.

Our thinking mind is an incredibly important part of who we are. The brain is the repository of countless memories, experiences, beliefs, feelings, behaviors, and character traits, all connected in a complex communication network. It's a huge storage facility packed with aspects of our identity. If everything that's stored in there forms your personality, who are you when you no longer have access to that storehouse where your entire life is kept? What's left of you when no new connections are made and no more information is transmitted about what you know, want, or like to do? Unless we really have to, we'd rather not think about it.

The word "dementia" is derived from Latin and literally means "without mind." It makes me think of the "dementors," the fictional creatures in J. K. Rowling's Harry Potter books. As the meanest, most hideous monsters in the entire series, they drain all happiness from the air around them. Those who receive "the dementor's kiss" lose their soul—it's sucked from their body, forcing them to live out their lives as physical, mindless beings. This terrifying specter feeds into our biggest fear surrounding dementia: that we may end up as an empty shell. I now know that this image doesn't even come close to describing the life of a person with dementia, but it's hard to explain that to someone who's had no first-hand experience with the illness.

We also look away from dementia and everything associated with it because of the widespread association with being labeled "crazy." Obviously, nobody wants to be thought of that way. I personally think it's not the most respectful term, but it's the word my mother used whenever we tried to have a conversation about what might be wrong with her. You should have heard her. "I'm not going *crazy*!" she'd snap, her dark eyes blazing, reducing the courage we'd plucked up to ashes. Did she feel watched and judged? To what extent was she aware that dementia was setting in? We can't say for certain, but what we do know is that she did everything in her power to avoid this particular label: To my mother, we were the ones who were crazy, not her.

EXONERATING

I'm sad to say that I, too, spent ages tiptoeing around dementia. Whenever the subject was swept off the table by my parents, by my mother's steadfast denial and my father's protective love for her, I'd drop it for a while, sometimes briefly, and other times too long. We all played our role in the family drama *We're All Just Fine*. Each act lasted until either my or my brothers' emotions ran so high and our discussions became so heated that we had to sit our parents down again and raise the possibility that something wasn't quite right with my mother's health.

"Mom, Dad, we think Mom might actually have dementia."

"Oh, come on guys, is this really necessary?"

After all this time, I'm still plagued by the feeling that perhaps I should have done more, that I should have insisted on answers. When my parents finally went to see their family doctor again, and only much later (too late in my opinion) received a referral to see a specialist, it didn't feel like a victory. It was but a temporary respite from our efforts. It's not as if we knew better than the health-care professionals. All we had to go on were snippets of a vague diagnosis. Every now and then I'd go online and search "symptoms of dementia" and "does my mother have dementia?" It would trigger a desire for more answers, but all too often I'd be swallowed up by my day-to-day life, and again we'd muddle along for a while longer. I know I'll have to come to terms with the fact that, like my parents, I allowed myself to be led by uneasiness and a lack of knowledge about dementia.

For a long time, I found it difficult to face up to the possibility of dementia, not just logically but with my heart and soul; to not only suspect it but to *feel* it. I remember an incident several years ago while having dinner with a few close girlfriends. The wine flowed, the food was good, and we were having a lovely time when one of them suddenly asked me how my mother was doing. I felt an icy-cold, leaden sensation in my stomach. How dare she? Leave my mother alone. That simple, considerate question caught me off guard. Admitting to myself that my mother was potentially, even probably, seriously and terminally ill was a difficult process for me as it was for my parents. Pretending that nothing was wrong was a temporary fix not only for them but for us all.

To make matters worse, I'm not the kind of person who takes comfort in figures and percentages and dry medical facts about dementia—that's simply not how I'm wired. Despite this, I still recognize knowledge as a way to make sense of what's happening to the person you love. I can say now with the benefit of hindsight that I don't know what I was so afraid of. It felt as if I had a stubborn little girl inside my rib cage, who'd sit there with her arms crossed, petulantly shaking her head every time "dementia" came up: *No*, not *my* mom. As if dementia would take note of such resistance. By the time my mother's dementia could no longer be denied, it was impossible to start over.

I wish I could write another story. In retrospect, we should have done things differently. This account of my mother's dementia isn't necessarily a textbook example of perfect management. What might a different past with an earlier diagnosis have brought? Perhaps we could have involved my mother more in the process of her illness and treatment (although I have my doubts about that). An early diagnosis helps you prepare for what's ahead and gives your loved one with dementia more time to think about and plan for the future.

Then again, to this day I haven't come across many people or stories in which the illness follows a clearly defined road map. An erratic, insidious beginning shrouded in chaos and confusion seems to come with the territory. Luckily, as a society, we're now more aware of this lack of knowledge and the associations that people who are not directly involved have with dementia. The more, and earlier, we hear that dementia isn't something to be afraid of, the better.

If you can, start your fact-finding mission today. You would not believe how many passages I underlined and forwarded to my father and brothers during the research phase of this book. My highlighters are nearly empty. "Look, we're not the only ones to have missed this," or, "See, the exact same happened to them!" It enables me to look at myself and my parents with compassion and see that there are *causes* and *reasons* why we went about things the way we did. Knowledge creates a clear and unprejudiced space in which what happened can be separated from feelings of guilt and blame. Maybe you're also looking back, thinking that despite your good and loving intentions, you wish you'd done things differently. If so, I'd like to bestow on you the powerful comfort of knowledge: *It exonerates.*

After a lengthy spell of home care, my mother moved to a care facility, where she's been living for the past few years. While writing this book, I had a few conversations with the social worker there about how we can engage with dementia in a meaningful way. Her work is best described as "dementia coaching," although that's not the official label. She supports the primary caregivers and the families of the day care patients and permanent residents, like my mother. This role gives the social worker her broad insight into what dealing with dementia means for the loved ones. I think the world of her because my father visits her regularly to express and come to terms with his emotions. My brothers and I have seen the positive effect this has had on him and his coping process. The first time I met her in her office—a wing of the building that smells of clean laundry and linoleum—she raised both hands mid-conversation and held them in front of her chest: "These are the two pillars of my work," she explained. "One hand stands for knowledge about the illness, about the nature of dementia; the other represents knowledge about yourself. How do you deal with setbacks and sadness? What lessons have you learned in life?"

I instantly understood which hand had been empty for too long. *That's* how important knowledge is: It's a foundation for the resilience and courage that you'll have to bring to the situation. Despite any resistance you may feel, it's vital that you learn what dementia really means.

Luckily, by the time I spoke to the social worker, I'd made up for lost time. I'd read stacks of books and trawled through countless websites to come to terms with the concepts of neurons and stacking proteins, loss of brain mass, and the role of short- and long-term memory. I'd read about treatment indications (which I still find incredibly complicated), social protocols, and the problems faced by primary caregivers. Wise and capable people from around the world have shared their knowledge about the practical, medical, and psychological issues you can expect to come up against in the direct care for and contact with your loved one with dementia. The many books about dementia for and by professional and primary caregivers made my eyes sting, but I do have a better understanding now. Immersing myself in that material has certainly made me more confident and compassionate toward everybody, including myself.

Now I'm saddling you with homework after all. I completely understand if that's not what you need right now. But trust me. As dry and brittle as the facts and details surrounding dementia may be, the "Oh, is that how it works?" moments can be life savers.

WHO ARE YOU IN THE FACE OF DEMENTIA?

Self-knowledge is one of the pillars of coping with the illness, and it includes your emotional well-being and survival. Maybe you feel uneasy about looking inward. Let's face it— you're not the one with dementia. Perhaps it feels downright selfish to turn to your own feelings, thoughts, and experiences when another person is ill. Isn't that . . . navel-gazing?

No.

Figuring out how you can maintain a sense of balance while also shouldering what may be one of the heaviest burdens of your life is essential. You must be mindful of the impact that dementia has on your life and discover who you are in the face of it.

In the beginning, the focus will be on the person with the diagnosis. The patient always comes first, as they should. But we can't deny that the condition affects you and others as well. Who has dementia, and who is impacted by it? It's not

PUTTING YOURSELF LAST ISN'T
SUSTAINABLE IF YOU WANT TO
KEEP BEING THERE FOR THE
PERSON WHO NEEDS YOU.

as simple as one plus one. Luckily, there's now a much greater awareness of dementia's effect on the patient's immediate surroundings, especially the primary caregivers, who take on an arduous role. Dementia doesn't just have an impact on the person who's been diagnosed, but on everybody around them, too. The Dutch psychologist Huub Buijssen wrote: "A chronic illness rarely affects just one person, and this is particularly true of dementia. Few illnesses cause such suffering among family members. That's why dementia has been referred to as a 'beholder's disease.'"

Modesty is admirable in the context of another person's suffering, but too much altruism will ultimately be detrimental to all involved. Putting yourself last isn't sustainable if you want to keep being there for the person who needs you. "I'll handle it," my father used to say, until he almost collapsed under the pressure of his singular devotion to my mother. "I was convinced I was strong enough to find a solution to every single problem and determined to take care of her. It was my job," my father would say. He ended up with severe burnout. My father's case isn't unique. As a daughter, I can tell you that whichever role you take on, you'll need all your strength. Without the healthy counterbalance of self-care and self-love, caring for someone can very quickly become isolating and draining. In her book *What Dementia Teaches Us About Love*, Nicci Gerrard captures that precarious balance particularly well: "The carer of someone with dementia lives between two grave dangers: of withdrawing in order to protect the self, and of becoming extinguished by the needs of the dependent other."

Dementia is a marathon, and one way or another we must find the physical, mental, and emotional endurance to make it through. Over time, both illness and caring become harder while anticipatory grief—grieving the loss of someone who's still alive—is an art in itself. Additionally, it's not as if you have a reward to look forward to or compensation for your dedication and care. Whatever you do, there won't be a happy ending. No fireworks, no balloons. It's not going to be all right or "work out somehow." You're doing it simply so that by the time it's all over, you're still standing and you can look back on a long and meandering road that wasn't just an endurance test.

It's a terrible cliché, but that doesn't make it any less true: You must look after yourself the way you'd look after someone else. It's the reason coaches and gurus always cite the example of oxygen masks on planes: Put on your own mask before you assist others. The metaphor is apt because you can only help when you have the ability to give. I hope you manage to make this journey work for yourself. Attending to your own needs certainly doesn't stop you from being fully there for another person. You should feel free to lavish as much care and attention on yourself as you would on your loved one.

Dementia is like a mirror that reflects back unfamiliar facets of your personality. My mother's dementia challenged me to know myself on a deeper level because she's counting on me. Self-knowledge helps you to keep going. It's useful to know how to charge your batteries and unwind, understand why you react the way you do, see what your fears and desires are, and think about which values your moral compass is set to. It helps to be aware of your strengths and weaknesses, what *truly* matters to you when it comes to decisions, and what you find comforting. If you want to be present, you must look at yourself honestly and objectively and hear your inner voice—that's authenticity. The deeper you're rooted in self-knowledge, the better you can withstand even the greatest storms.

The person close to you with dementia will benefit from your loving self-care. You can only offer calm, patience, courage, and resilience when you have a consistent source to draw from. You can be immensely useful to your loved one with dementia *precisely* when you're also tending to your own garden, pruning, weeding, and watering the flowers. I refer to my inner world as "the garden in my heart" because everybody understands that gardens need regular maintenance.

Simple exercises for boosting self-knowledge

1. Reflect. Look back on your life and ask yourself how you reacted to major changes or stressful situations in the past. What held you back and what helped you? What would you have done differently?

2. Make a list of the ten inner values that are most important to you. Next, cross out five. Then another two. You *have* to choose. The three remaining qualities form your inner compass. They'll always point you in the direction that matters to you, making future decisions and deliberations easier.

3. Alone time is important. Give yourself a daily moment to be alone with your thoughts. This can be difficult when you're the primary caregiver and you have to be alert at all times, but you can also use activities like dishwashing, folding laundry, or grocery shopping to check in with yourself. How are you? What do you need?

4. Keep a simple diary and jot down how you're feeling and what's having a positive and negative effect on your mood and energy. Do this long enough and you'll discover patterns.

SELF-COMPASSION MATTERS, TOO

While we're on the subject of the self—self-knowledge, self-insight, self-care, self-examination, and self-love—I'd like to say a few words about *self-compassion*. It belongs in the medicine cabinet of the soul, and you're going to need regular doses of it. One of dementia's best-known and nastiest side effects for beholders is the constant nagging pain that the work they're putting in is *never enough.* This sense of falling short, dropping the ball, taking the wrong turn may seem unavoidable. For me personally, the sentiment is all too familiar. For example, on one occasion, my father phoned in the middle of the night, but I was unable to go and see him because as a single mother, I couldn't leave my young children alone. Nicci Gerrard's observation in *What Dementia Teaches Us About Love* is very relatable.

> For surely the endeavor—the never-quite-possible endeavor—for a carer is to tread the quicksand strip of middle ground between the abandonment of the self in the name of love and duty and the unyielding protection of the self in the name of survival. To both give and keep hold of the self, to accompany the person who is leaving while also staying behind. . . . They will always feel that their work is never good enough. Guilt floods in—guilt at being human and having desires and needs of one's own. Health and survival can come to seem like acts of infidelity: to have a space for oneself a betrayal.

You can walk this tightrope between self-sacrifice and self-preservation with the help of a balancing pole. Self-compassion is a safe and reliable aid. Putting it into practice helps you re-center yourself and return to the center of your gravity, the point at which your equilibrium is restored, even if only momentarily.

Kristin Neff, a leading expert in the field of self-compassion, identifies three elements of it: self-kindness, common humanity, and mindfulness. Being kind and understanding toward oneself is often the opposite of what we do when we feel a sense of inadequacy or failure. "What did you do *that* for?" or "I'm no good at anything!" whispers the angry little voice inside my head when I handle something badly or I can only visit my mother briefly. We go from bad to worse with the addition of guilt and shame. Why are we so hard on ourselves? You wouldn't use that tone with a child or a good friend, would you? Treating yourself the way you'd treat somebody dear to you is self-compassion in a nutshell. It may take a bit of getting used to, but being kind to yourself is simple yet incredibly powerful.

Nobody is perfect, and we make mistakes so we can learn from them. We all slip up from time to time, and sooner or later we all face setbacks. That's what Neff means by "common humanity": Recognizing that you're not the only one who's suffering or making mistakes has a soothing and comforting effect. Nobody is guaranteed a carefree life; worrying is part and parcel of our time here on earth and it's what makes us human. I strongly believe in the compelling sentiment that "sharing our hurt is sharing our humanity."

Finally, Neff highlights the importance of mindfulness for self-compassion. Mindfulness is the art of observing your emotions as they are, without judgment, pushing them away, or wallowing in them. It starts by acknowledging that you have feelings, but that you are not your feelings. Buddhist teachings capture this in a classic metaphor: The emotions you feel are like the clouds, the rain, the sun, and the mist moving across the mountain. Who are you in this analogy? You're the mountain, not the weather. It's a good thing to remember when you're having a hard time.

You can practice self-compassion whenever love encounters pain. When you're dealing with dementia, this happens all the time and you'll have ample opportunities to practice, whether you like it or not. Thupten Jinpa, a former monk and longtime principal translator of the Dalai Lama, has written a beautiful book about compassion, *A Fearless Heart*, in which he defines the concept as "a sense of concern that arises when we are confronted with another's suffering and feel motivated to see that suffering relieved." He goes on to say: "Compassion offers the possibility of responding to suffering with understanding, patience, and kindness rather than, say, fear and repulsion. As such, compassion lets us open ourselves to the reality of suffering and seek its alleviation." Compassion literally means "suffering together." The "self" merely serves to remind you that it's okay and natural to have compassion for yourself, too.

Don't confuse self-compassion with self-pity. When you feel self-pity, you're more inclined to disconnect your own experiences from those of others. With your focus turned inward, the internal space in which you experience those emotions becomes smaller and stuffier. Self-compassion, on the other hand, throws open the doors: It gets the air circulating and creates room and a sense of connection. It makes the resistance to "what is"—in this case having to bear a loved one's dementia—less oppressive and suffocating. It lets in the oxygen.

Self-compassion equals forgiving, accepting, and being kind to yourself

Here's how to practice:

1. Don't put yourself down. Words are powerful, including the ones you whisper to yourself. You're not "stupid" just because you did something wrong. You're not "selfish" because you need a break.

2. Don't rush to say "sorry." All too often, we apologize for things that aren't our fault. Instead of "sorry," try saying "thank you." "Thank you for waiting for me," "Thank you for letting me tell my story."

3. Forgive yourself. Write it down on a piece of paper or say it out loud in front of a mirror: "I forgive you."

4. When you notice that you're being hard on yourself, ask what you'd do for your best friend—then do this for yourself. Draw up a list of your best qualities, the skills you're most proud of. Appreciate how unique they are, both in this particular situation and in combination with your personality and path in life. Think of the moments when these qualities will stand you in good stead as you face someone with dementia.

5. Acceptance doesn't mean approving of what happens to you or no longer caring about it. It means accepting that you can't change it.

6. Begin more sentences with "It's okay to . . ." (rest, start over again, have moments of carefree fun, be at your wits' end, ask for help, feel what you're feeling, or rethink a decision, to name a few).

THE FOUNDATIONS

WHEN YOU MEET ADVERSITY IN LIFE

The following three concepts are useful as you walk the path of dementia: coping mechanisms, the five stages of grief, and the family soul. These are just a few of many insights and resources, but I believe they will provide an easy and accessible route toward a better understanding of yourself and those around you. They'll certainly come in handy while reading this book.

COPING MECHANISMS AND HOW THEY WORK

Have you ever spotted a solitary fisherman by the side of a lake, staring at his rig? It may as well have been my middle brother. A few years ago, he took up fishing again, and now he will occasionally leave his hectic job and family life for a quick break, chuck his rod into the back of the car, and drive to the water to gather his thoughts. At the same time, my elder brother may be getting on his racing bike, which he'll mount on an indoor trainer at home and sweat his way through the many hard miles that his cycling coach tells him to complete. My father, meanwhile, will be somewhere photographing a statue, landscape, or lunch-for-one on an outdoor terrace before sending his photo to the family group chat. *Ping.*

And me? I write.

The word "coping" can mean "handling," "enduring," "surviving," and "managing." In essence, "coping mechanisms," a term used in psychology, are the ways in which people choose to deal with stress, anxiety, and disappointment. These are caused by external difficulties that cross your path (such as bad news or challenging situations) or by distressing thoughts and feelings that bubble up from within. Often the two go hand in hand.

How one deals with tough situations and unpleasant feelings varies from person to person. We all have a unique set of coping mechanisms for getting through off days: our own "coping style." Your personal toolkit may contain one or more of the following: withdrawing, frantically searching for solutions, denying that anything is wrong, taking your anger out on something or someone, or buying yet another pair of shoes.

A coping mechanism isn't necessarily bad or something you need to unlearn; there are plenty of healthy ways to make adversity more bearable. Just think of the relief you feel after a nice long walk to clear your head or following a meal with a good friend. Less advisable tactics involve pouring yourself that extra glass of wine, snapping at a supermarket cashier, or obsessing over inconsequential details. These defensive behaviors are not coping mechanisms but rather clumsy forms of self-preservation, ways to avoid owning your feelings or doing what needs to be done.

Your coping style is shaped by what you learned when you were younger, what you've taught yourself during earlier setbacks, what you're used to, and how much you can handle. Maybe you've never thought about this, so I'd like to emphasize that there's no "good" or "bad" way of dealing with dementia. We tend to handle situations the way we do because we haven't found a better alternative. Just as we have our own reactions to the diagnosis, we have our own ways of coping during the illness.

Some mechanisms offer sustainable and positive support whereas others are best seen as temporary solutions in an emergency. It's good to distinguish between the two because ultimately, you benefit most from a more supportive style. Why don't you take a closer look at your mechanisms and divide them into two piles: "helpful" and "unhelpful"? You can even write these down the old-fashioned way, using paper and pen. I do this when I feel stressed, agitated, or overtired and it helps me learn how my coping mechanisms affect the situations I'm in. Are you feeling lighter now that you've done the exercise?

If you want, you can add a third pile: "*could be* helpful." Positive coping mechanisms can be identified and learned. They can become valuable stepping stones that form a bridge between stress, anxiety, and tension on one side and renewed energy, health, and relaxation on the other. What it boils down to is this: Positive coping mechanisms foster well-being, negative ones don't. It's useful to remind yourself of this when you encounter obstacles on your path.

Examples of helpful coping mechanisms

1. Expressing your emotions in a way that feels safe

2. Talking to others about your feelings and experiences, perhaps in a dementia support group

3. Making up for your weaknesses by practicing something you're good at

4. Processing your emotions through physical activity, such as walking or another form of exercise

5. Drawing on your experiences to help others or to bring about positive change

6. Gathering information about what's worrying you; knowledge can create clarity and a sense of control

7. Noticing everything that's going well

8. Engaging in mindful activities, such as drawing, doing jigsaw puzzles, gardening, and cooking

9. Spending time in nature

10. Keeping a regular diary

11. Making small, loving gestures toward yourself, such as having a cup of your favorite coffee in the morning or using a fancy shampoo

Examples of unhelpful coping mechanisms

1. Denying that anything is wrong
2. Running away from the situation—physically by being out a lot or mentally by ignoring the situation and your emotions
3. Consuming too much of something: food, sugary snacks, the internet, your phone, alcohol, or cigarettes
4. Fleeing into your own fantasy world
5. Idealizing everything that's going well to cover up what's not going so great
6. Projecting your feelings of powerlessness onto others by lashing out at your nearest and dearest, caregivers, or even "the whole system"
7. Rejecting a diagnosis or the assistance of others
8. Willfully breaking rules, like speeding or ignoring directions
9. Using narcotics, such as sleeping pills
10. Ploughing on and never relaxing
11. Lacking initiative or saying "no" to everything
12. Letting humor give way to cynicism and sarcasm

THE FIVE STAGES OF GRIEF

Dementia is sometimes described as a long, drawn-out process of grieving. Saying goodbye while your loved one is still alive is the stark reality of this disease. When I talk about dementia, I often compare it to a trapdoor that could open at any time and send us hurtling down yet another floor. On each new level your loved one has lost a little bit more, be it the ability to form sentences, find the bathroom on their own, or raise a fork to their lips. You notice it, yet you need to keep going. You have no reason to mourn, as the person you love is still physically with you, yet you're grieving. It's a quiet grief.

When you're mourning a loss, however great or small, someone will draw your attention to Elisabeth Kübler-Ross's five stages of grief. Many grieving people have felt seen thanks to these acclaimed phases, as they offer validation as you find your way through the dark forest. Kübler-Ross, who died in 2004, developed her take on palliative care and mourning during her work with terminally ill people, including patients living with HIV/AIDS in the 1980s.

The model doesn't cover everything and isn't without its faults. The experience-based findings have never been substantiated by scientific research. Nor are they absolute—they're based on a Western form of mourning, and for that reason alone, they are not universal. Kübler-Ross later expressed regret that people interpret the stages as a step-by-step guide to the "correct" way of grieving. She highlighted that there's no such thing as a road map for grief. Everybody goes through the stages in a different order, and you can't just check them off. You may find yourself going through the same stage more than once.

That being said, I find the five stages valuable. By labeling and defining recognizable "states of being," they provide a degree of support. They pluck you from a fog of emotions, even if temporarily, and ground you again. These are the five stages.

Anger

"What has life thrown at me now?" At this stage you feel anger, perhaps even aggression. Irrationality is never far off. We don't prize these emotions highly in this Western corner of the world; they're at odds with self-control, decorum, and the idea that life can be shaped. Anger is one of the purest emotions, one of the primary human responses. The beauty of anger is that it's like fire: You can use it as fuel, but stoke the flames too high and you run the risk of burning yourself and causing irreparable damage.

Bargaining

You want to put up a fight and put your back into it instead of accepting this reality lying down. The energy that's released at this stage is conducive to bargaining. People who are forced to come to terms with a loss may make emotional decisions with significant consequences during this phase. Perhaps they opt for a radical change in lifestyle, set ambitious goals, or make grand, bold resolutions: "I'll never give up!" The bargaining is aimed at taking matters into your own hands or changing fate. It's an "If I do this, then . . ." negotiation with the cosmos, a transaction: If you make a promise, then surely you can expect something in return. You try to wrest back control just as forcefully as it was taken away from you.

Denial

"Don't worry, she's just absent-minded" and "Tomorrow we'll be back to normal." Denial is often our first response when we realize something is wrong. It's a subtle trick that our mind plays on us, seeking to protect from a painful truth that may be too big to take in all at once. By refusing to accept reality, you can keep living on autopilot a little longer. Survival and staying afloat come first. Children do this when they can't process news right away: They'll blink a few times and continue playing, only to suddenly burst into tears later in the day. Reality can simply be too overwhelming for us to wrap our heads around.

Depression

Then comes the realization that our struggle is real and there's nothing we can do about it—anger, resistance, denial . . . none of it helps. All roads ultimately lead to the same outcome: reality as it is. It unleashes a wave of powerlessness and sadness. This despair has many faces: Some people turn inward and become apathetic and distant; others become visibly emotional. To make matters worse, it's not uncommon for unprocessed trauma to resurface along with new grief.

Acceptance

Acceptance is also referred to as "adjustment." It's not that you resign yourself to what's happening but rather that you reorganize your life around the loss and see reality for what it is. A degree of acquiescence sets in. Some reach this stage sooner than others, and sometimes a period of acceptance will be temporary until a new trapdoor opens.

THE FAMILY SOUL

Earlier, I wrote about dementia being described as a "beholder's disease." Most of us are not alone in caring for or worrying about someone, as each person with dementia often has many supporters. There's a hierarchy, with the patient and primary caregiver at the center and widening circles of intimacy around them. It's rare for any of them to play the same role or to see things from the same perspective. While one may be responsible for handling practical matters, others may do their caring from a distance. Either way, there will be a number of people who are in some way regularly involved with the person with dementia over the course of their illness.

In my family's case, my father was the primary caregiver for a long time, and he's still the one who spends the most time with my mother now that she no longer lives at home. He visits her practically every day. Then there are my brothers and me, followed by my sisters-in-law and the grandchildren. Others include my aunts and a few of my mother's close friends. Finally, her caregivers have now also become part of her inner circle. All these stakeholders form a galaxy with my mother as the central planet; closer or further away, in smaller or bigger orbits, we revolve around her.

Dementia really lays bare the intricate network around the person with the condition. It will be much clearer to you that you're not the only one whose opinions or actions matter. Within the family, each individual has one or more roles, be it a partner, child, parent, brother, sister, aunt, or uncle. All these stakeholders bring their own hopes, sorrows, values, and desires to the process and have their own views and emotions. This marks the start of a complex choreography that will sometimes have you moving forward and other times taking a small step back while being careful not to tread on too many toes or encroach on anyone's space.

It's important to recognize and acknowledge this system and know you're not alone: we're all in it together. As you read earlier, we're all at different stages of grief and have our own ways of staying resilient. We're not synchronized swimmers moving in the exact same way to the rhythm of the music; we're just splashing about, trying to keep our heads above water and often end up accidently hitting each other.

All of us have been part of a family system all along that predates the dementia. How we respond to events that happen to us in our adult lives is deeply rooted in how we were raised and which values were consciously or unconsciously passed on within the family. Much of your emotional makeup was instilled in your early childhood, which means that the collective you're a part of isn't just something external to you: It forms the core of your being, like the rings inside a tree, and continues to shape how you react to tension, stress, or grief.

Not reverting to old patterns, sharp criticism, or unspoken expectations within your circle of stakeholders is another challenge in times of worry. Those who are interested in personal growth and self-development will likely be familiar with this inspirational quote from the spiritual teacher Ram Dass: "If you think you are enlightened, go and spend a week

AS A FAMILY, YOU'VE
FORMED A COLLECTIVE SOUL,
WHICH CAN BE PASSED ON
FROM GENERATION
TO GENERATION.

with your family." Its implication is clear: Being the best, most "enlightened" version of yourself is probably hardest when you're with your own family.

Maybe you learned to shout just a little bit louder than everyone else as a child to be heard, or the opposite: You're always trying to keep the peace and don't mind putting your own needs on the back burner. Perhaps you're the clown who likes to inject a note of levity into the proceedings, or you're someone who's not used to talking about emotions because no one at home ever did. It's easy to slip back into these behaviors when you're facing intense challenges together. In these difficult circumstances, dementia can lay bare the fault lines within a family.

The family system is also referred to as the "family soul." As a family, you've formed a collective soul, which can be passed on from generation to generation. It's a gentler take on the idea of a galaxy we're all orbiting in. The concept of the family soul represents something that may be less immediately apparent, but certainly palpable. I once heard it described as the wind you can't see, except in the leaves of the trees dancing on it. "We're a tenacious lot" can be an unconscious family motto, or "We cherish our independence." There are more problematic variations, too, like "We don't talk about our feelings" or "We're not weak." All are mottoes that influence how you relate to one another or handle situations. Your family soul can color everything you do and think as an individual, and you're often not fully aware of it.

The family soul or the idea of a collective isn't something negative or oppressive. In fact, when caring for a loved one brings old dynamics to the surface—and it almost always will—you may grab this moment to bring about change, and maybe even start a process of healing and connection.

It's fair to assume that everybody wants only the best for their loved ones, despite how clumsy, ill-advised, or wrong their approach may be. Not every person will feel the exact same way at the exact same moment. However, all people ultimately have one goal in mind: minimizing suffering and discomfort and maximizing love and well-being. I recommend you reread that line when someone says or does something you don't understand or approve of because it will clear the air and make space for compassion. The dementia that you all are collectively dealing with may be a good opportunity to try to get to know each other better, reflect on how things have been in the past, and how we might change that in the present.

It's encouraging to consider how a family system can develop and transform over the years. This may not be the right time to sift through your family system in detail and resolve *everything* that's going on—quite simply because there's something more urgent that demands your attention—but taking care of someone with dementia together gives you an opportunity to consider how you and your circle demonstrate curiosity, kindness, and compassion. I frequently ask myself the question: "Is what I (or what others) want *better* or just *different*?" And if I'm being honest with myself, it's often the latter of the two.

You can't change your family single-handedly. Faced with dementia, there will always be moments of misunderstanding, irritation, and even anger toward the other caregivers, but you can make a positive contribution by doing whatever you can to change the way the wind blows. You don't have to radically shake things up—soft power can get you far. Why not be more forgiving, practice compassion, and give each other space? Be prepared to see the good in other people's actions and intentions. Don't project your expectations onto those around you, but be grateful for what you're achieving together.

We are one another's caregivers, too. As family, we must give comfort and support and be there for one another. As Ram Dass said: "We are all just walking each other home." We must continue to look after each other, making sure that nobody falls over or is left behind. Dementia is lonely enough as it is.

THE CHALLENGES

FACING UP TO PAIN AND SADNESS

Not long before my mother was admitted to a nursing home, my parents moved. By the time they started looking for a new place, my mom hadn't been her usual self for some time. Although initially opposed to moving, when she saw this apartment, she enthused about its view across the water—we took that to be a "yes." The idea that they selected this place *together* is one of those little things we clung to, perhaps against our better judgment. This was our mother's choice, too—at least that's what we told ourselves. It's why my father had her blessing to feel at home there.

We'd hoped they'd continue to live together for a while, free from insurmountable staircases and spare rooms gathering dust. Her name is still on the sign by the door, but things didn't go as planned. My mother would get out of bed at night, refusing to go back to sleep. She'd lose her temper with my dad, loud enough for the neighbors to hear. She mulishly turned away, chair and all, whenever the home help aide came. Her dementia became erratic and unmanageable.

In the end, she only lived there for a few months.

It would be naive and unrealistic to write about dementia without mentioning the huge wave of complex situations and agonizing moments that wash over you in its wake. Of course, all the attention should first go to the person with the illness—that goes without saying. People with the condition can be scared, angry, fearful, and ashamed during every stage and continue to have these emotions throughout the process, except they'll be harder to predict, decipher, or explain. All you can do, as a loved one, is look on, and that makes you feel powerless and sad. If only you could remove the many challenges, but you can't—at least not in any significant way. You often end up pushing away your own difficult emotions. In the light of another person's suffering, you may feel inappropriate or simply too much.

It's perfectly understandable why people around the patient slip into survival mode and put their own difficulties on hold, but dementia also triggers feelings in you, which there's no use ignoring. Being attentive to your feelings may not feel like a priority; it may even feel selfish. Yet your pain isn't a cross to bear out of guilt or shame. It's *impossible* to leave your own emotions at the door; you take them wherever you go—they'll be in the room with you while you care for your loved one.

And let's not forget: You have every *right* to feel what you're feeling. Caring for and about somebody with dementia is exhausting, raw, and intense. Loving someone makes that pain more acute. Looking after and worrying about your loved one with dementia can bring you to your knees, pull you back up again, and push you to (and beyond) your limits. There's no road map to guide you around deep troughs and along sharp bends, no manual for dealing with this condition. The very least you can give yourself is the permission to embrace your own humanity.

In an interview with a Dutch newspaper, Edith Eger, a psychologist and Holocaust survivor, said: "It took me a long time to understand that pain doesn't disappear when you run away from it; that only makes it worse." She went through hell to learn this life lesson that everybody has to internalize in their own way: that difficult circumstances benefit most from our full attention, from the bright light of day.

Difficult emotions are indicators, directing our attention to what matters most. They form part of the inner compass that shows us the way, and as such they're just as important as positive emotions. We must look pain straight in the eye to understand what it wants from us. In fact, we need feelings like shame, fear, and anger because they keep us on our toes and get us to act. From a purely evolutionary standpoint, they're essential for the survival of our species. However painful they are, they're a natural part of being human. Ignore them and they'll only keep clamoring for attention. It may sound paradoxical, but giving difficult emotions their proper place will make your life lighter. Acknowledging what you feel allows you to stop fighting against yourself and begin to embrace who you are now, with everything that involves, including pain and sadness.

But perhaps you don't want your emotions to become lighter. Sometimes we resist letting go, be it consciously or unconsciously. As counterproductive as difficult emotions may be, they form a link between you and the person you love. By feeling them, you'll keep their presence in your heart alive and kicking. It's something I recognize: There are times when I *enjoy* feeling sad. When my eyes fill with tears because I wish my mother could be with me, it feels as if I'm honoring her, as if I'm letting her be part of the moment. I cherish those tears.

There's certainly no need for difficult emotions to be resolved or exorcised. All that matters is that you can let them in, and then let them go again. That's what feelings are for. A child who trips and falls will burst into tears, but at some point they'll be over it. They will get up again and continue playing.

Don't let all the pain, sadness, and feelings of powerlessness sink to the bottom of your heart. Let them float to the surface, where you can identify and study them and find out what they're trying to tell you. The poet Rumi summed it up wisely: "The cure for pain is in the pain."

It's also important to admit and acknowledge emotions because you may experience burnout or depression as a result of suppressed pain and unprocessed trauma, especially when combined with the tough responsibilities of being a caregiver. The combination of keeping your head above water in day-to-day life without noticing and taking the time for your own feelings is toxic. Loving primary caregivers buckle under this heavy weight every day. You can only carry it for so long.

The cover of this book promises words of comfort. Maybe that got you hoping that we wouldn't be talking about the challenges that dementia brings. But I believe in the healing power of recognition and acknowledgment, in drawing attention to the rough edges. Sometimes we must move toward our greatest fears and shine a light on the things we don't want to see. Facing up to the cause of our pain and sadness takes courage, but when we learn to show up for the process of dementia—including all the pain, shame, and grief—we can genuinely connect with others who suffer. That alone brings understanding and space, however contradictory it may sound. The realization that you're not alone in what you're feeling, experiencing, and thinking is one of the magical ingredients that comfort is made of. The decision to neither numb nor suppress your emotions but to confront them head-on is empowering.

And do you know what's encouraging? Feeling these emotions is a sign that you're okay, that facing up to life is something you can handle.

SHAME

When my father reflects on the difficulties of living with my mother's illness, the conversation often turns to two major emotions that have troubled him and continue to plague him: shame and guilt. He's not alone. These feelings are etched deep in the hearts of everybody who loves somebody with dementia. My father told me this story: "When it began to dawn on me that your mom was getting worse and I was having to take on more care responsibilities, it took me a long time before I was able to tell other people—aside from you guys and a few others who were really close to us. Every week I'd drive to choir practice with a friend, and every week I'd be sitting next to her in the car, wondering . . . should I tell her *now*? That my wife is very ill, needs more and more care, and is becoming less and less independent. Every single week I was determined to say something to my friend. I'd wanted to tell her, 'I can no longer manage on my own and I'm going to need your help when all our partners come along on a choir outing.' But I didn't."

It was shame that was stopping him.

I think shame is one of the most complex emotions to handle. It's easily blown out of proportion and won't readily be reduced to a manageable size again, like an air mattress you're trying to stuff back into its original packaging after use. "Shame," in the broadest sense of the word, is often defined as the acute feeling of discomfort we get when we don't conform to the rules of a particular group. And we see ourselves or our situation through the judging eyes of people in that group. It's the sense of not being able to comply with prevailing norms, of not fitting in, of being excluded. To smooth out this wrinkle between yourself and the outside world as quickly as possible, you'll naturally try to hide anything that's out of place or quickly divert attention to something else.

My father has plenty of anecdotes about the shame he's experienced: shame about my mother's growing lack of independence and the awkward situations they'd find themselves in while out in public. On one occasion he accidentally pressed the alarm in the disabled bathroom of a museum while helping her use the toilet, and on another he was standing on one side of a ticket barrier with the train ticket and she was on the other, struggling to understand his instructions. He could feel people's eyes boring into them. It breaks my heart to think that I wasn't there, but I appreciate that my father and I can talk about it now. Shame is something we *have* to discuss. In her bestseller *Daring Greatly*, Brené Brown writes, "If we *speak shame*, it begins to *wither*." Shame gains traction in silence and loses strength when we express what we feel. Precisely because shame is about feelings of exclusion and isolation, the antidote is connection and recognition. The writer Nakeia Homer also encourages us not to hide or cover the things we're embarrassed about: "Someone else will be *inspired* by the part of your story you're ashamed of." It's a comforting thought.

While learning to handle my mother's dementia, I also felt shame. And shame multiplies with shame about the shame. I wish I could write that it wasn't so. In the early years of my mother's illness, I was often embarrassed by her. We weren't sure whether she had dementia or not, but we knew something wasn't right. She hadn't been herself for years. I remember making small talk with store clerks, trying to distract them from my bumbling mother, while irritably taking my mother's wallet out of her hands. At birthday parties I'd keep an eye on her, worried that she'd get caught up in awkward conversations or otherwise flounder in social situations. Sometimes I'd feel ashamed on both my parents' behalf, because my father would compensate by doing the talking *for* her—always speaking in terms of "we," never "I"—and my mother would stand there, nodding meekly.

As someone with early onset dementia (my mother was only in her sixties when the illness began), she had to cope with additional challenges. She looked youthful, which created an even bigger gap between her mental well-being and her physical exterior. For a long time, you couldn't tell that she had dementia. If only I could travel back in time and look at her more lovingly and help her during those moments. She must have felt so helpless during everyday life. But I didn't know, and she didn't know, and shame wormed its way in.

The fact that shame and dementia are so closely intertwined has everything to do with the ignorance and fear I described earlier. Not fitting in is the essence of shame, and it touches on the fear of being seen as crazy, of having people whisper about you: *Is this woman not quite in her right mind?* It's the fear of not being taken seriously, not being recognized as a full-fledged member of society, but standing out and being judged on an illness that's befallen you. It's like living inside a bell jar, isolated from everybody else.

Although we're talking about our shame and way of dealing with dementia, we mustn't lose sight of the heartrending fact that it's the patients who are at the center of all the unwanted attention. When it dawns on somebody that they're losing control over themselves and can no longer shoulder the responsibilities they once took for granted, it causes a great deal of pain and sadness. It's that shame experienced by both the patients and those around them that's behind many of the early problems. There might be a delay in seeking a diagnosis, or else it will be rejected, along with the necessary support, which in turn puts an extra heavy burden on the (primary) caregivers. It's worth bearing in mind, however, that not every patient is aware of their condition. With those who have frontotemporal dementia, for example, a refusal to accept what's happening is an integral part of the illness. That said, shame still plays a role in that difficult first phase. My mother didn't want to know about our concerns, because her strong sense of autonomy and her reluctance to stand out simply wouldn't let her.

The loss of autonomy generated recurring feelings of shame for my father, even after he'd stopped being her primary caregiver. He told me: "I was ashamed to say to strangers, 'My wife doesn't live with me; she's in an assisted-living facility.' I also felt terrible when I had to sign documents on her behalf. I was ashamed of having a spouse who was incapable of giving her own consent. Autonomy is incredibly important to me, and I would have loved to have her beside me as the strong and independent woman she used to be. That was my wish. The moments when this was so obviously *not* the case filled me with shame. I wanted her to be fully part of the world. And she no longer is."

It's comforting to know that the shame eases over the years. My own lessened as my mother's dementia advanced. It became crystal clear that there was a cause, a reason for everything that made her different, and that there was nothing she could do about it. Now I feel less of a need to explain her actions when I see puzzled faces and prying eyes staring at us in public. The shame has disappeared, creating more space for compassion and self-confidence.

It's strange to think that the dementia I've railed against has also become the bridge across the shame, a bridge toward her, because now the illness is simply a fact. These days it's no longer an issue for me to go outside and walk by her side, with her sitting quietly in her wheelchair and me singing to keep our spirits up. Passersby are treated to a friendly smile. I don't mind feeding her small bites of cake, giving her something to drink through a straw, reading to her, ignoring her loud teeth grinding, or combing her hair, all without any pinpricks of shame.

Unfortunately, advancing dementia can't always completely remove shame (or milder embarrassment). The inappropriate and inconsiderate behavior of someone who suffers from a loss of decorum, for instance, will always be at odds with our ideas of what's "normal" and "decent." Dementia can make people act in ways that are difficult to witness: removing their clothes for no reason, urinating in strange places, using obscene language, yelling, swearing, or other aggressive behavior. The father of a dear friend of mine began to make sexist remarks to his caregivers—it's uncomfortable, whichever way you look at it.

Maybe there's comfort in seeing shame in a different, more loving light. I've come to realize that the shame I felt for my mother's dementia was in fact an awkward expression of my love for her. Like my father, I was ashamed not because I thought she was stupid but because I wanted her to be her full self. I longed for her to be the strong woman she was (and is), without being overshadowed by the dementia.

You're ashamed because you love someone. You're ashamed because you want only the best for that person. You're ashamed because the reality is at odds with the dreams you cherished for yourself, for them, and for you together. This is known as "empathic shame." It's shame born of love, of our ability to empathize with another person. Shame is rooted in empathy and compassion, in our wish to provide our loved one with social safety, to defend them against criticism or exclusion. The more we care about someone, the more acutely we feel this urge to protect.

When you feel the burn of shame, why not leave it burning like a candle on the altar of your love?

GUILT

"If we take her, she won't be coming back home." These are the words of the case manager sitting on my parents' sofa. My mother is in bed with severe delirium. It's the culmination of weeks, maybe even months, of increasing worry. Her health is going downhill fast. Aware of the gravity of the situation, we nod patiently. We all know that we can't continue like this, with my mother at home, despite my father's unending sense of duty, despite the home help, despite all our best efforts. This bladder infection that has sent her into an acute state of confusion is the final straw. The situation has become untenable. My mother needs round-the-clock specialist care, both now and after her delirium, and my father is completely worn out.

It brings a tsunami of responsibilities. Where we live in the Netherlands we need to obtain the correct care assessment and find a facility that will accept her, then pack up her medication and pajamas. I look back on those days and weeks as a tangled mess of panic, sadness, guilt, and powerlessness.

Once we'd found an emergency place where she could convalesce, my aunt and I got her out of her bed at home for the last time. "We're going for a drive," I lied to my confused mother, and together we ushered her out the front door, knowing that she'd never set foot in her own home again. That moment still grabs me by the throat. The rest is a bit of a blur: the waiting car, the nursing home, an impersonal room that we decorated with a wooden ornamental bird from the apartment. Doctors, examinations, tears all around. If he could have, my father would have taken her straight back home again, in the trunk of the car if necessary.

That time when I led her out of her own home isn't the only moment when I felt like a treacherous Judas. The lowest point for me was the assessment. In the Netherlands, there is an institute, Centrum Indicatiestelling Zorg (CIZ), that assesses whether someone is eligible for long-term care and if the costs will be reimbursed. My mother hadn't yet received assessment for the facility that had promised us a place after endless phoning, pleading, and begging. Her emergency home, a residential nursing facility, had music by a jazz trio every Sunday and chairs made of the softest calfskin leather, but she would sit there all alone in the living room, and I rarely saw any of the caregivers. We really wanted to get her out of there. The care home we did like was a gift from heaven because they specialize in early onset dementia. However, the one barrier was the compulsory care law, which prevents involuntary admission. My mother would have to consent to long-term admission.

It is decided that my elder brother and I will talk to my mother and the lady from the CIZ. My father is completely exhausted, so my other brother will be staying with him. Our meeting is in the conservatory at my mom's temporary home. The windows have decals of birds, we have a view of the woods, and our mother is sitting between us on the sofa. Anyone looking in would think we were enjoying a pleasant visit together, but we know better—we're here to get our mom to consent to a future she doesn't want. It's crunch time. She *has* to say "yes." The stakes are high: If she doesn't agree, her place in the nice care facility could go to someone else, and we can't stomach any of the alternatives. My brother and I *must* pull this off.

I feel sick, like there are strobe lights flashing inside my head. I'm having an out-of-body experience; it's as if I'm hovering above the scene like a drone. I can see myself, my mother, my brother, the CIZ lady.

"Mrs. Helmink, do you understand that the ward will be locked, and that you won't be able to come and go as you please?" The woman goes on and on (she's only doing her job, I know, but I feel like slapping her).

"Ma'am, do you consent to admission?"

"*Ma'am?*"

My mother's dark eyes flit from my brother to me, helplessly, flashing with bewilderment. She's having difficulties talking, but eventually stammers "Yes." Her fate is sealed. The CIZ lady closes her folder and leaves. I manage not to be sick.

My elder brother, my rock, my hero, breaks.

I've never seen my brother cry like this.

Coping with dementia is steeped in guilt. Whatever you do, it's not enough; it will never be enough. The best choice is a measly lesser of two evils. It's a minefield of "what-ifs" and "if-onlys." Have I done enough? Could I have done something different? What if we'd opted for B instead of A? As Huub Buijssen writes in *The Simplicity of Dementia*, "Feelings of guilt often take little, or no, account of what is reasonable. They whisper to us that we could always have done *more*."

Beside the difficult choices we had to make on my mother's behalf, I also felt torn between caring for her and the many other things that demanded my attention, like my children and my job. It wouldn't have been feasible to just drop everything and be with my parents day and night. They certainly wouldn't have wanted me to. Guilt is the IV we're all hooked up to; every day, it slowly drips into our consciousness. Whichever place you occupy in the care hierarchy, this sense of falling short or playing catch-up will gnaw at you. Primary caregivers get the worst of it, as the guilt can stem from resistance and powerlessness, feeling *forced* to care by circumstances and a sense of duty.

Whatever their source, feelings of guilt chip away at our quality of life. Anyone who feels they're not good enough will always live with a degree of self-rejection. Hugely demoralizing, it can manifest in the body in the form of physical pain, like a cramp. There's a reason that people speak of feeling "weighed down" by guilt. As my father puts it, "I kept telling myself, 'I can do this. Whatever happens, I'll find a solution.' I was convinced I was strong enough to deal with any problem and to keep looking after her, just as I'd promised. 'Oh well, we'll pull through,' I'd think after every setback." Unable to honor his vows to her, not even with all the will in the world, my father collapsed under the weight of his sense of duty. The moment that my mother had to leave home because caring for her had become too hard was when the guilt pulled the rug from under his feet, and he really went to pieces for a while.

Guilt is a downward spiral that seldom leads to positive change. When you can't cut yourself some slack, whether in the form of time for yourself, rest, or relaxation, you end up recharging less. Caregivers tend to set the bar too high on what isn't a level playing field to start with, and the dementia is always going to win. You can never do enough, and that's a tough reality to face. My father had to abandon his vow to look after my mother "in sickness and in health," and that broke his heart. He had to get back on his feet, learn that he's allowed to have carefree moments, enjoy the beauty of life, and go forward without her always by his side.

This quote by Huub Buijssen also got me thinking about guilt and why we feel it.

In cultures in which everything is believed to be predestined, as in India for instance, feelings of guilt do not exist. We Westerners, however, believe strongly that our own efforts really do make a difference. Without feelings of guilt, life would be one big game of chance, including our contracting—or not contracting—a fatal illness, our own capacities, the moment of admission to a nursing home, and so forth. We cannot believe that, and we do not want to believe it. Behind every feeling of guilt there is an almost child-like feeling of power, the thought that there is a tiny piece of God in all of us. The psychological purpose of guilt, therefore, is that it drives us to control our own lives; and because we need to do this so badly, feelings of guilt can be very persistent indeed.

His words make me wonder whether our feelings of guilt may be misguided. It's humbling to realize that as people we're simply not powerful enough to change or influence the reality of dementia. Our sense of guilt stems from expectations about control and ideas about our own influence. The idea that if we work hard enough everything will be all right is rather cruel. Once we come to the humbling conclusion that we don't pull all the strings and that not everything is possible if we try our best, much of that oppressive responsibility is lifted off our shoulders, and our sense of guilt eases a little. Ultimately, accepting our feelings of guilt means accepting our powerlessness.

Self-compassion helps you do this. I must have muttered "I'm doing what I can" a thousand times. It doesn't remove the guilt completely, but it does transform it from a massive burden into a fluid energy that will help you keep showing up and keep going as best you can. I wish the alleviation of this guilt for my father, my loved ones, you, and me.

We mustn't be under any illusion that guilt can be reduced to nothing. The social worker at my mother's care facility stressed this during one of our conversations, explaining: "There will always be a bit of guilt, but maybe that's not a bad thing. Feeling guilty is an expression of your love. For example, you'd wanted to look after your loved one at home for longer, and it hurts that you couldn't do so. When you view your guilt in that light, in the light of your love for and great loyalty to the person with dementia, it's actually something special. Why not embrace it? It's a way of expressing that you care."

LIVING AWAY FROM HOME

This feels like the right place to address the dilemma of having your loved one live at home versus admitting them to an assisted-living facility, a nursing home, or other form of residential care. This dilemma is closely tied to feelings of guilt and falling short. In fact, I've noticed that people speak of "saving" their loved one from the nursing home as the pinnacle of altruism and kindness.

Obviously, I can't comment on the best housing for somebody in a particular situation—that's highly personal and dependent on a great many variables—but creating a hierarchy in care options just isn't fair. Such preconceptions about good and bad and the best way of dealing with dementia are of no help to anyone.

We shouldn't be blind to the fact that living at home until the very end simply isn't for everyone. There are too many complex medical, financial, and social factors at play to adopt a one-size-fits-all solution when it comes to dementia care. Surely we can't saddle a caregiver with additional guilt because they can no longer make the home situation work. It's nobody's fault; it's just the dementia mapping its own uncompromising path.

In June 2021, Judith Bom, a health scientist, completed her doctorate with a study of the impact of nursing home admission and the role of primary caregivers. One of her key findings was that people are no worse off in a nursing facility than they'd be in their own home. In the final stages of dementia, it makes no fundamental difference to their well-being. But those who *are* noticeably better off are the primary caregivers, who have an onerous burden lifted from their shoulders and are finally given the space to prioritize their own well-being again. This research provides an interesting alternative perspective and reflects my own experiences.

While we may not have saved my mother from the nursing home, the nursing home did save us. My mother lives in a nice place, where she's sheltered from the outside world and can relax with her symptoms. Instead of having to function in a world that's too demanding and overstimulating, my mother is now somewhere that's set up for her dementia and where there's always someone to look after her. I've seen my father change from an overworked primary caregiver back into her husband, her pillar of strength. Most days, my father will get there in the morning and they'll listen to music together. The staff often makes him a sandwich, too, as he practically lives there and they're moved by my parents' close bond. This is another way for two people who love each other to be together. After all those years of unconditional care, he no longer needs to prove his love by caring for my mother at home.

Not all nursing homes are the same, and there's plenty of room for improvement. In the Dutch care sector, for example, there should be more intermediate setups that bridge the gap between living at home and admission to care, because the transition is often too abrupt. I'm not blind to that; we've been through it ourselves. But I'd like to assure you that it's not all gloom and doom. I know lots of people whose loved ones, like my mother, live in a pleasant and safe place.

Ignorance and fear of what dementia is and what dealing with the condition involves means that people are sometimes needlessly denied a form of care that would be good for them. Sure, the linoleum in my mother's facility isn't the best, and yes, sometimes you can smell the incontinence products— some people happen to be wearing them. At the end of the day, do those initial impressions really matter?

I challenge you to look beyond them. My mother is cared for in a way we couldn't have provided ourselves; she's safe and she's seen. She's surrounded by attention, knowledge, and expertise in her nursing home. I've accepted the fact that she no longer lives in her own home. Of course, I wish the situation were different, but then again, I wish *everything* were different.

ANGER

I got a phone call at work. It was my father, and he was panicking—my mother had disappeared. My parents had taken my young sons to the historical village Zaanse Schans for the afternoon. One moment Mom had been waiting on a bench while Dad and the boys climbed one of the windmills and waved at her from the top. The next minute she was gone. I jumped in my car and made my way over to the tourist attraction, while the park rangers and the police went in search of my missing mother. Just as I pulled up with screeching tires, she was dropped off in a patrol car. She got out, looking surprised. She'd walked out of an open-air museum and had been found at a gas station miles away. My boys were given a sticker by the police. The color gradually returned to my father's cheeks. All's well that ends well, right?

Everything was fine.

Well, no—this isn't the end of the story.

In a daze I joined my relieved father, confused mother, and two happy children at the Zaanse Schans. Now that I was here, my father said, I might as well stick around. We looked at sheep, cottages, and windmills, and ate ice cream in the sun. When we finally did make our way to the exit, a park photographer had his camera at the ready. "Cheese," my father said, and we had our picture taken. I got into my car with the children and drove back home. But with each mile we covered, I began to tremble more and more. Not with shock (OK, maybe that, too), but with anger. I flew into a rage—for the first time I became uncontrollably angry.

I wasn't angry because my mother got lost. Nor because my parents kept doing fun stuff, even after my brothers and I had expressed our reservations about taking my mother on outings. It wasn't about any of that. I was angry because of what happened *next*: Business as usual. Oh well, my father thought, now that I was here I might as well have a look around, too. It was ridiculous and absurd, and something in me snapped. I was livid—with the dementia, with my father, with everything and everyone, including the farce in which I'd been allocated a role, yet again. When I look back on it now, I think that's when it dawned on me that the house of cards was falling, that the dementia was about to drastically disrupt our lives. Had my mother *really* just been found outside a gas station by the police?

I thought everything was fine?

Of all the difficult emotions, anger isn't my favorite. Admitting to anger is difficult; I prefer to call it "sadness" or "confusion." And yet sometimes pure rage rears its head. Giving that emotion an honest, open place when dealing with dementia is a challenge. It doesn't really fit the puzzle. Who are you meant to be angry with? What do you aim your anger at? Nobody is to blame for the situation as it is, least of all your loved one. Self-control appears to be the only option.

But let's face it: There's plenty to be angry about. Anger is the painful check you're presented with after a generous serving of sorrow, disappointment, powerlessness, and fatigue. You're pushed too far or too hard or both. Rage is a very pure, natural response to the tidal wave of injustice that washes over you. You've been forced to give up so much: your carefreeness, your time, the well-being of someone dear to you, future dreams, your life as it was. As a (primary) caregiver, you sometimes feel like a prisoner of your own life. Day in and day out, everything is determined by the other person's dementia. It holds you hostage, while everybody else seems to be worry-free. Is it any wonder that it feels jarring at times?

My father doesn't show his anger much, but not long ago it suddenly slipped out. My brother and I were chuckling about something, but he took it as a bored reaction to something he'd said (which wasn't the case). "I *know*," he said in a real huff. "I'm repeating myself! But this is my life! Every morning I get back in the car, park outside the nursing home again, play the same old music in her room, sing the same old song.

On a good day, she'll give me a smile, or a kiss. On other days, she barely notices me and doesn't show much joy, and I'll be driving home with the knowledge that that's my lot for the day. This is my life!" We were surprised, but also relieved: Go on, Dad, let it all out. We were strangely pleased that for once he poured his heart out to us. We have to let go of the taboo on expressing exasperation and frustration in this way, that anger is a sign of weakness. The opposite is true: It's a powerful "no," a way of pushing off against the bottom of our emotions and finding our way back to the surface again.

There's every chance that your anger will be aimed at your loved one with dementia. I'm sure that almost everybody, certainly in the initial stages of the illness, has reacted sharply to someone close. In those early days, especially, it's difficult to figure out why suddenly things aren't going smoothly anymore, why somebody can do something one day but not the next, or why you're not getting an answer to a perfectly clear question. This unsettling behavior provokes irritation; in fact, annoyance will simmer throughout the entire illness. You'll hear unfinished, incoherent stories; witness fumbling with routine tasks; find yourself keeping a constant watch on someone; and having to rearrange your own plans over and over again. The behavior caused by dementia can get on your nerves—there's no two ways about it.

Under "normal" circumstances, you'd deal with your frustration by talking things through or by being more vocal about your expectations or wishes. But when somebody has dementia, you can't have that kind of conversation on an equal footing. You can't in all fairness blame the other—that would assume they could change or improve. And if the person picks up on your irritation or resulting anger, it often makes the atmosphere more strained, because they won't understand why you're angry. The result? More confusion and uncertainty.

Bottled-up anger is like a powder keg: It takes only a tiny spark for you to explode. You don't want that, because there's no healthy place for anger in a care relationship in which one person depends on the other. Another regrettable side effect of pent-up anger is resentment and bitterness, so it's important to find an outlet. When you notice your anger and frustration building into utter despair, don't hesitate to ask for help to avoid exploding. You wouldn't be the first to be at your wit's end. Perhaps tensions are already running too high. If so, I wish I could pull you through this page and give your tense body a big hug. Please share your feelings. You're not being unreasonable. You're human and vulnerable.

As with all difficult things, the safe release of anger always begins with acknowledging that you're angry. It begins with giving yourself permission to feel the emotion, just as it is. You can ease the tension and rid your body of some of the pent-up energy by moving around. Stamp your feet, snap a branch in half, throw pebbles into the water. Shout at the wind, or inside your car—nobody will hear you. Grunt, clench your fists, and relax them again. Punch your mattress. It all feels uninhibited and unsettling, but that's the point.

When you're calm again, you can reflect on your anger. You might want to figure out what your triggers are. What's making you feel so angry? When do you feel it well up within your body? Maybe the muscles in your back are tightening, your pulse is up, or you're feeling flushed. Perhaps your breathing is shallower. These are all cues to take a deep breath, literally count to ten, or walk away from the situation if it's safe to do so. After a while you may be able to detect a pattern and break it by doing or planning something different or getting help. It's good to have a clearer idea of where your limits are and when you come up against them.

Finally, you can ask yourself whether your anger is trying to tell you something. Maybe you're not angry, but sad. Or scared. As the expression goes: You can't see your reflection in boiling water, just like you can't see reality reflected in anger. Sometimes anger masks what's going on at a deeper level. It can be a distraction, a kind of pose you adopt to protect yourself from the real pain.

DENIAL

The story about the family outing to Zaanse Schans, along with the anger I felt back then, are closely tied to the frustration that built up during the lengthy period when my parents were in denial. However lucky I am with my father and brothers, that first phase of my mother's dementia left us all feeling ragged. We look back on that time with mixed feelings, and I think I'm also speaking for my brothers when I say that much of our shared grief can be traced back to the term "denial"—masking, avoiding, concealing, and misrepresenting the elephant in the room.

For my mother, the topic of dementia was off-limits. She'd physically turn her back to you if you so much as mentioned the words "diagnosis," "screening," or "support." It was probably caused by the condition itself; understanding is rare in patients. My ever-loyal father wanted to protect her and was fighting a battle on two fronts: with my mother and with us, his children, who kept pushing for more clarity and openness. Because we couldn't really blame my mother, our growing frustration was directed at my father. I was exasperated by his cloak of undying love, while equally moved by it. I sympathized, yet because that cloak covered absolutely everything, I sometimes didn't feel seen or heard in my own worries and grief.

But what we didn't know at the time, and what my parents didn't realize either, is that we were following in the footsteps of other families affected by dementia. My parents' behavior was far from unique or deliberately obtuse. They didn't do it *on purpose*. Dementia patients will do anything they can to put up a smoke screen and hide the incipient illness. It's so common, there's an official term for it: "confabulation"—unintentional lying about events or fabricating or exaggerating in order to mask reality. Realizing that you have dementia and understanding what that condition is doing to you are two separate things—and in many cases patients can't do either. People with dementia genuinely don't know what's happening; at best, they'll sense that something "isn't right."

Because it's highly likely that this denial is caused by damage in certain parts of the brain, even at this early stage, there's not much point in thinking you can make a difference by having a constructive conversation. While those of us with a healthy brain go into a process of recognition by talking, acknowledging, understanding, and accepting, this is something that a person with dementia is probably no longer capable of. It's also the reason why support services soon turn to those around the patient, particularly the primary caregiver. Often, they're the ones who'll have to do the work of acceptance and facing up to reality.

That said, the patient's (primary) caregivers are just as likely to go along with this denial. For them, it's a coping mechanism, a way of not having to feel the grief that dementia brings. Let's pretend everything's fine, and then we'll see what tomorrow brings. Nicci Gerrard describes this dynamic in *What Dementia Teaches Us About Love*: "People who care for the person who has dementia—above all, if they are their partner or spouse and have built up a relationship of mutual affirmation—often collaborate with them in this task of confabulation. After all, they have been taking part in the same performance for so long, a double act and each other's audience. Carers give their loved ones alibis, cover for them, finish their sentences, take up the stories they are telling, explain them to others, even join in with the stressful pretense of normality." My father would print out synopses for my mother's book club, because she thought they were "really handy." He seemed oblivious to the fact that after years of devouring book after book, she was suddenly incapable of finishing one. Bit by bit, she became more dependent, while he didn't think twice about stepping up to the plate. Before they knew it, they were walking down the path of confabulation together. "I did it all without giving it too much thought. I just liked being able to help her," he says about it now.

Looking back, I have so much more understanding and compassion for what he went through. Besides, it's not completely unfamiliar to me. There were times when instead of confronting my parents I agreed to "leave it for now," because it was the summer vacation, or nearly Christmas, or we were having such a nice time together. I'll be the first to smooth over differences and make sure everyone's comfortable. Sometimes it was easier or more convenient to temporarily park dementia in the underground garage of my consciousness, so I could see to routine business at ground level.

In other words, denial and avoidance are common ways of dealing with stressful events. They're forms of self-protection, ways of temporarily pushing away a painful realization. The more you love someone, the more blurred the boundaries between the self and the other become—and by denying something you're not only protecting yourself, but also the person you love and your life together. It's our mind's clumsy way of staving off the reality of a situation that evokes resistance. It's not the same as lying, which is deliberate denial or misrepresentation.

We all do it from time to time; we're all guilty of denial in some shape or form—turning a blind eye to something we don't want to know about, looking away to protect our fragile heart and our sensitive soul. But when denial becomes a long-term strategy, it no longer places a soft, protective shield between the self and reality, but a towering wall instead. You're going to need ever more tricks up your sleeve to uphold that alternative universe.

When denial is no longer an option, there's only one alternative: accepting the fact that in the coming years, you and your loved one are up against a long and messy illness with an inevitable conclusion. Letting this fully sink in, knowing there's no hope of a different outcome, is a tall order. It's no wonder that we'd rather close our eyes to that brutal prospect while we can. In her book *Dementia Essentials*, Jan Hall says, "From the outside, denial can look as silly as the ostrich's mythical 'head-in-the-sand' reflex, but from the inside, that denial may simply be the last line of defense against just giving up. . . . Do you really want to take that away?"

For a long time, my father found himself painfully torn between avoiding the label "dementia" and facing up to what was happening. He protected their joint line of defense with fierce commitment. He later said, "Your mom didn't want to talk about it. You guys kept bringing it up. I was caught in the middle. But if I'm really honest with myself, I must admit that I was only too happy to pretend that maybe things weren't so bad."

There can be no denying my mother's dementia anymore. That phase is well and truly behind us. My father's denial, though not completely gone, has turned into a somewhat gentler wishful thinking. He hasn't put away his sparkly magic wand and likes to see reality in the most glowing, most positive light. He still struggles to accept difficult things and is knocked off balance every time she's sad or withdrawn during a visit, has lost yet more independence, or when the doctor has bad news. He tends to look at my mother's situation through rose-tinted glasses, and he still likes nothing better than to huddle with her beneath that heavy but warm cloak of love. I no longer blame him—it's what he needs to do to keep going. When my mother appears to be smiling, he can go home with a spring in his step. The slightest indication that she's calm and content will get him through the day. It's fine. We let him have his magic.

Why would you want to take that away?

The common thread running through everything that's difficult is grief: grief for what was, what is, and what's to come. Grief for what the other person is going through, as well as a more muted grief for your own life, which is taking a different turn from what you'd hoped or planned. Grief is very good at hiding. It can disguise itself as anger, fatigue, or apathy, and sometimes it's veiled by optimism or obscured by distraction. But ultimately it underpins everything. Nicci Gerrard writes, "I know that I have variously described my father as a great ship untethered and slipping out to sea, a town whose lights are going out one by one, a bombed city, an ice floe breaking up and becoming smaller and smaller until there is no place left to stand." That's an image that can only be evoked by raw, unadulterated grief.

Unlike other emotions, grief can be very elusive. It can feel rarefied like air and solid like a clod of earth, it can burn beneath your skin like fire and surge through you like water. "Time heals all wounds," we tell ourselves, or "It will pass." But in reality, it doesn't work that way. Grief is never "done," at best it changes shape. When you enter a new phase of life, it feels like you're back to square one and you have to weave it back into where you are and what you're going through at that moment.

I experience my grief like a silver thread that connects me to my mother. Grief is sometimes described as love with no place to go. Love that can't be reciprocated. As I get older, I keep feeling the grief in new ways. I've spun a thread from it and woven it into my heart—that way she's always with me, living *within* me. When I imagine running my fingers across my heart, I feel it's textured, that it's no longer as unblemished as it once was. That's her. And it comforts me, strangely enough.

My father lives according to what he calls his "80/20 principle": "80 percent of the time I'm able to maintain my equilibrium and 20 percent of the time I'm out of kilter. This 80/20 principle has become my way of life. I stick to it, because the grief I feel in that 20 percent is my love for your mom. I'm not aiming for 100 percent, because I wouldn't be doing my relationship with her justice."

He takes an emotional pause.

"I *have* to feel the grief. I've integrated it into my life and know that it will affect me from time to time. I might be walking around the house, crying, and then I'll think to myself: I'm dealing with my 20 percent now. It does me good in a way. It's cathartic. If I didn't let that grief in, I'd feel as if I were leading two different lives: one during the hours I spend with her, the other doing my own thing and enjoying life. I can't do that. I need my grief to be able to set about the other 80 percent again. I want to feel the pain because I also feel the love in it."

"WE HAVE TO BE ABLE TO BEAR SORROW—NOT TO TURN AWAY FROM IT, NOR TO ABSORB IT OR ENTER INTO IT, BUT TO BEAR IT. SORROW IS A HEAVY WEIGHT."

—*Nicci Gerrard*

"But Dad, it still pains me to hear that. I would love for you not to have to bear that grief," I say to him.

"I don't want that. I'm fine like this, with my 80 percent. It's my balance."

Feeling sad and feeling strong aren't necessarily at odds with each other. I came across a beautiful quote from the writer John Green that really touched me: "Grief does not change you. It reveals you." It's true; grief reveals your heart and soul. By doing so, it also brings about something beautiful and pure—a way of staying close to yourself. No, time doesn't heal all wounds. It's what you do with your grief during that time to make your life more authentic and more truthful. It's about making space for all the grief, both the huge sorrow of losing someone, saying goodbye, and letting go, and the little sorrows of seeing yet another memory carried off by the wind. None of it will simply dissolve, but we can bear it if we bring kindness and tenderness to it. As Nicci Gerrard puts it, "We have to be able to bear sorrow—not to turn away from it, nor to absorb it or enter into it, but to bear it. Sorrow is a heavy weight."

There are ways of getting to know your grief a bit better. You'll discover that grief doesn't run on a schedule; it comes and goes as it pleases. Nor does it have a script. It always unfolds in its own unique way. Some people prefer to process grief alone, in isolation; others can cope with it only through the warmth of human contact. Some need more time than others to find a way to live with it. Perhaps you've been made to feel that you're not supposed to be sad for too long, or too visibly or too intensely. But there's no "right" or "wrong" way to do grief. People are allowed to help, comfort, or advise you, but they must never take your grief away from you.

A problem with grief in our culture is that it often comes with an unspoken hierarchy. We draw circles of grief around the person with dementia: The partner comes first, followed by any children and/or parents, next are the brothers and sisters, then the rest of the family and friends. It conceives of grief as something that you have more or less of a right to or that you can measure. But there's no such thing as a unit of grief, the way we measure weight or height. You can feel a huge amount of compassion for another person's grief without it diminishing yours in any way.

Grief is colored by your character, life experience, religious or spiritual views, cultural background, and more. That's what makes it personal and unique to you. At the same time, grief is a universal human experience, with one and the same source: love. We all feel grief, but not all in the same way. That's why imposing a hierarchy of grief won't help you or others—it leads to alienation at a time when we really need to connect.

When grief washes over me, I don't suppress it. I may be talking with my father or brothers about the past, or about how my mother is doing, and then suddenly the tears start flowing. When that happens, we don't make it any bigger or smaller than it is. We just let it be.

FEAR

It's not unthinkable that you'll develop feelings of fear as your loved one grapples with dementia. It's no surprise: Now that everything you've always taken for granted has changed, your world has become less safe and more unpredictable. A major setback or an intense experience automatically puts you into a state of alert. What else should you be afraid of? This constant, often subconscious, vigilance is exhausting. It makes your muscles tense up, slows your thinking mind, and heightens your emotions. While fear *feels* like a warning of something that's to come, it's often a reaction to something that's already happened.

There are many ways to deal with fear. It helps to talk about your emotions with someone you trust, which unscrews the relief valve and releases a bit of tension. Knowledge is always useful, too. It will exorcise demons, as fear is best friends with fantasy and the imagination. To calm your hyperactive nervous system, try to be mindful of your breathing. Your breathing will often be too rapid and shallow when you're tense. As soon as you notice irregularities, breathe slowly and deeply, in and out through your nose, letting the air fill your belly. Consider going for a walk. Moving your feet has a calming rhythm that will enable your body to rock itself back to a sense of security.

Because the relationship between fear and dementia is so multifaceted, I've broken it down into three distinctive forms of fear.

Fearing the world of dementia

One year, on National Volunteering Day, I joined the editorial team of the magazine I worked for to help out at a home for people with learning difficulties. Many had been there since childhood and had been institutionalized for much of their lives. Some of the residents had reached the age where they were also developing dementia, which made their behavior particularly hard to gauge for someone who doesn't encounter it every day. When my babysitter canceled, I was forced to take along my younger son, who was about three at the time. I didn't think it would be a problem. A cheerful and friendly child, he happily stepped into the circle of residents and my colleagues and shook everybody's hand. Until, that is, he reached one of the residents . . . and had a shock. He quickly withdrew his little hand and ran crying into my arms.

It was so upsetting to me at the time. Like any parent, I want my children to meet the world with an open mind, without judging anyone on their behavior, appearance, or intellectual abilities. I hope my kids can see through those things, and I try to set a good example for them. I was reminded of the incident years later, when my mother moved into her residential home, and I noticed that, although my children are older now, they still find it daunting and a little bit scary to come along. They can't really read the people with dementia. Some will move their faces very close to theirs and ask weird questions, or else make silly noises and generally not behave in a "grown-up" way.

Even *I* feel uncomfortable at times as I make my way to my mother's ward. Whenever something unpredictable happens or I hear a scream that cuts to the bone, I'm on the alert. When a male resident keeps walking right behind me in the corridor, I end up feeling a bit anxious, too. I want to be mature and strong about it—I *know* it's no big deal—but he's a big, tough guy and I'm not always sure how to judge a situation or act in the right way.

Fear of the world of dementia can become particularly acute when your loved one starts attending outpatient care or moves into a permanent facility. Visiting means stepping into that world. Every time I tap in the entry code and the sliding doors open, it's like entering another dimension. You'll find a broad spectrum of people with dementia here. Some residents are still of reasonably sound mind and may be sitting at a table playing cards, while others are in the later stages of the illness. You hear sounds you're not familiar with, smell odors that are new to you, see situations that aren't easy to read.

Maybe you're someone who has no trouble crossing that threshold. It's no longer a big deal to me, but I know people who still struggle. Fear of unpredictable and confrontational behavior can have an inhibiting effect on the frequency of contact. When you recognize that this fear is impacting you or someone close to you, it may help to visit together or look for other ways to remove some of the barriers, such as meeting in a neutral location, like the yard or cafeteria.

In her book *Dementia Essentials*, Jan Hall explains, "Some people are good visitors, and some are not. Some feel awkward, as though they need reassurance from the person they're visiting that it's worth their being there—and that reassurance does not always come." Her advice: Approach a visit like a project, prepare in advance, and evaluate afterward. What went well, what less so, and how might you handle it on a future occasion? She cites the example of a man who kept a diary of his visits to his dad—not to document the progress of the dementia, but purely to record the interaction with his father and the positive experiences. I thought it was a great idea. My visits to my mother have greatly improved since I've started preparing better. Now I always bring a book to read to her and something to eat. In the car on the way home, I identify the most positive aspects of our time together and keep them in my heart.

Fearing your loved one's advancing dementia

Aside from the fear of losing my mother, I've also been apprehensive about what the dementia is doing to her. In my mother's case, the illness robbed her of language early on. Aphasia, a speech impairment caused by damage to the left side of the brain, severely hampers communication. There were times when she was inconsolable. While we may have had a medical explanation, these episodes remained very difficult to deal with. At times I was scared to enter her room. What if she isn't having a good day? What if I can't get through to her or comfort her? What if she has needs that I can't help her with? What if I'm missing something? My mother's inexplicable sobbing was distressing because it made me feel powerless.

Dementia can trigger a wide range of behaviors, including the unfiltered expression of emotions, deep-seated suspicions, and a loss of decorum. Some people with dementia scream or yell, others are aggressive or anxious, and yet others burp loudly or hide valuables in strange places. Behavior can be as changeable as the weather: One moment all appears to be fine, and the next there'll be an outburst without any apparent cause. When my mother still lived at home, there were times when she'd cry uncontrollably. Often our fear has nothing to do with the behavior itself but with our perceived inability to handle it. It's no surprise, then, that you'd rather steer clear of such stressful situations. The unpredictability of dementia makes them difficult to navigate.

Dementia will eventually lead to physical deterioration, and that can be frightening, too. It's not always easy to talk about. Someone's appearance may alter, for example, because they stop looking after themselves, plus the body's motor skills change. My mother's posture has transformed completely, as has her facial expression. She grinds her teeth, a damaging tic she can't seem to shake, and sometimes she'll reach for things that I can't see, which is unnerving. And while you know intellectually that it's "part of the process," emotionally it can be a very different experience. Decline can look and feel strange and trigger fear for the future. You don't know how fast the dementia will advance, and how much more the body and mind will degenerate. This unpredictability, this volatility, robs you of any sense of control. And when medication comes into the picture, especially in the later stages of dementia, you may feel that you can no longer read your loved one correctly. You wonder if they need more medication, or less? Can you talk to a medical practitioner about it, and if so, how can you make the right decisions together?

When your loved one moves out of the family home, a perceived lack of control can become acute. You're no longer there to witness every moment and you're forced to rely on caregivers. Do they know which perfume she likes to wear? Do they know which music she prefers to listen to? Will they notice when she's in pain or hungry?

Maybe you worry about missing key moments or important information and losing any last vestige of control. That, too, can be a fear that will have to be managed.

Fearing one's own incipient dementia

"This is it," I message my brothers. I attach a screenshot of an email I sent to a coworker about a planned meeting. The subject line read "Thursday, August 25." In the body of the text I wrote, "Can you make Tuesday, March 15?" It wasn't until my colleague emailed me back that I saw that the dates didn't match and made no sense. I have no idea what was going on in my head—I thought I'd checked my schedule. Every time I forget a word, can't think of a name, fail to remember an incident, or say "spoon" when I mean "fork," I feel a jolt of fear: Here we go.

In my case, there's no real reason for this fear. While my mother may have early onset dementia, it appears to be an unfortunate twist of fate. It doesn't run in her family, and her own mother, my grandma, is still alive, well into her nineties, and mentally as sharp as a tack. That should give some genetic consolation, at the very least. That said, heredity can certainly play a role in passing on dementia. You can get tested for it, but as with all hereditary conditions, testing is a complex, personal choice. We didn't see any reason to have such a test done.

Dementia is thought to be the most widely feared health condition, even more than cancer or a heart attack. As I mentioned, the illness is surrounded by a great deal of anxiety and preconceptions. The fear of developing it is compounded by the fact that it's unclear if and how it can be prevented, and that there's currently no cure. Rational or not, I know the fear of dementia is acute among primary caregivers, who must be extra alert while caring and therefore feel especially dependent on their mind.

This fear of falling ill can be a heavy burden on top of all your other worries. That knot in your stomach when you've lost your keys, feeling your heart in your throat when you find your purse in an unexpected place, the hyperfocus on all manner of little signs that suggest that something isn't quite right—it can all be emotionally exhausting.

But there are ways of putting this fear into perspective. It's good to know, for example, that a certain degree of forgetfulness is normal. The older you are, the more often you'll forget something. If you're taking certain types of medication or if you're experiencing increased levels of stress, a higher workload, or hormonal changes, you may also find yourself forgetting more than usual. That's true for all of us—not every memory lapse is a dementia diagnosis waiting to happen. If you can't think of a word, forget what day it is, or something slips your mind, it's worth remembering that people who develop dementia aren't usually aware that they're forgetting things or making mistakes. Often, the reactions of friends and family give them their first inkling that something's wrong. It's usually the nearest and dearest who start to worry long before the one who's forgetful or displaying awkward behavior. In other words, while you're still hyperaware that your memory is letting you down from time to time, there's every reason for optimism.

Then there are certain lifestyle choices, which experts believe may help prevent dementia. Most of these will be familiar to you, because they're the usual tips for a healthy life: no smoking, moderate alcohol consumption, regular exercise, a good body-fat percentage, a varied and wholesome diet, and social interaction with other people. All this is good for your brain. Avoiding long-term stress and keeping your mind agile (for example, doing puzzles or learning new things) is also thought to lower the risk of dementia.

In practice, it can be hard to change your habits and comply with all these guidelines just to prevent something that's uncertain and far in the future. A textbook lifestyle can feel like an extra burden when your loved one's dementia demands all your time and attention. But being kind to yourself and taking little steps in the right direction is always better than nothing. Each apple chosen over a bar of chocolate, each glass of wine not poured, and each walk taken are positive changes.

FATIGUE

The day-to-day practical cares and intense emotions that come with dealing with dementia can result in a fatigue that doesn't go away with a few extra hours of sleep. The caring and worrying, the physical, mental, and emotional exhaustion can make even the simplest, most mundane tasks feel like you're swimming through syrup.

It's no surprise that you're tired. When all your energy disappears down a bottomless well, you may feel that you're no longer yourself, that you're spent. That's what I used to experience every time I drove away from my parents' house or my mother's nursing home. I'd be overcome by a deep emptiness, with muscles like jelly, a head full of fog, feeling completely burned out and used up.

Anyone going through a tough time should see their energy as sacrosanct rather than an afterthought. We think it's perfectly normal to plug in our phones when the battery is low, yet we're surprised to find that we feel drained when we don't take time to recharge ourselves. We mustn't dismiss "recharging" as navel-gazing or a waste of time.

Consider the following options: (a) falling over, or (b) staying firmly upright. Which do you choose?

Ha, it's a trick question! The person who instinctively opts for answer B is most at risk of ending up in scenario A. Being tired isn't a big deal, but you need to discover what you can do to stop yourself from becoming overtired.

Recharging

Here are some tips that might inspire you to incorporate brief recharge moments into your daily routine.

1. Close your eyes for fifteen minutes, either sitting down or standing up.

2. Switch your cell phone to silent or airplane mode for fixed periods of time.

3. Go to bed an hour earlier.

4. Choose ease over effort every now and then (order in food, have your groceries delivered, etc.).

5. Allow yourself to do something that isn't necessarily "useful."

6. Take a 20-minute power nap.

7. Use essential oils, such as lime or mandarin oil.

8. Take a warm shower or bath to relax your muscles.

9. Breathe with your hands on your lower abdomen.

10. Massage your wrists and hands or other pressure points on your body.

11. Walk barefoot.

12. Listen to running water.

13. Wear soft, loose clothing.

14. Make a to-do list to download practical matters out of your system.

15. Eat green leafy vegetables and fresh fruit.

16. Brush your hair or treat your skin with a nice lotion.

17. Create a quiet corner in your home.

18. Cuddle a loved one or a pet.

19. Write in your journal.

20. Hold your head lower than your heart (adopting the child's pose in yoga, for example).

21. Roll a tennis ball under the sole of your foot.

22. Stare into the distance without fixing your gaze on anything.

23. Sit or walk in natural light.

ASKING FOR HELP

"Dad, why did it take so long for you to admit that the two of you couldn't cope on your own?"

"If I accepted help, I had to concede that I could no longer manage by myself—whereas I *could* look after us both. Or so it seemed. I knew I dropped the ball from time to time, but I kept thinking, all right, I'll buckle down and deal with it somehow. Until I got to the point where I started dreading each new day. I'd be pacing up and down the living room, at my wits' end. I started calling you guys at all hours because I simply didn't know what to do."

For a long time, asking for help and receiving support remained sensitive subjects for my parents. It was difficult to make them see that we had to get some form of assistance, even if only around the house. We arranged for domestic help and private agencies to send somebody over to sit with my mother while my father went out, but it wasn't exactly warmly received. It was only when my mother began to become confused at night and when her frequent crying fits during the day left her withdrawn that my parents' defenses began to crumble under the weight of the advancing dementia.

We can't cope on our own—my parents can't, we can't, none of us can. That's one of the biggest lessons I can share from this experience. In my family, we missed out on a chance to act sooner, like so many others in our position. Asking for and accepting help requires vulnerability and openness, both of which are at odds with the desire to protect and maintain one's independence. It's a complex maze that's not navigated lightly.

But the stakes are high. In the short term, it's not easy to allow other people into the crude reality of life with dementia. In the long term, however, it's vital. Unless you admit others, loneliness awaits . . . along with the heavy burden of nonstop responsibility and alertness, physical and mental problems due to not having enough me-time, loss of social contacts, and blurring of boundaries between what you want to give and what's sustainable in the long term. As a caregiver, you're entitled to support. Perhaps not according to the letter of the law, but certainly according to the universal laws of compassion.

To this day I'm sorry that my mother so stubbornly rejected any offers of help, and that my father was determined to go it alone. My mother, especially, couldn't get herself to accept assistance; her character and the dementia made for a volatile mix. Had my parents become accustomed to support and outside visits at an early stage, both of their lives might have been easier. Seeing another familiar face, that of a professional caregiver or home health aide, for example, can be invaluable during the later stages of the illness.

"I can manage on my own" sounds noble. Coping alone is shrouded in a weird kind of heroic aura. The ability to shoulder a heavy burden is a sign of discipline, productivity, and composure—qualities that are directly linked to "success" and "status" in the Western world. In individualistic societies like ours, people are raised on the idea that if you work hard enough, you can be in control of your life. We're brought up to derive a certain sense of self-worth from the burden we can carry. Wow, you're so strong, you're so *independent*. Sure, it's satisfying to achieve, solve, or create something on our own, which boosts our confidence. There's certainly nothing wrong with stepping up your efforts for a set period of time. But ultimately these efforts must be proportionate to your downtime if you want to provide long-term care.

Perhaps you recognize the following. You don't ask for help, because

- deep down you're convinced that your way is the only right way,
- you think it's your duty to take care of the other person,

- you simply never learned that you're allowed to call on others, and
- you were taught that you should never "owe" anybody.

There's an alternative to being so independent and strong. Asking for help or indicating that you can't do it all by yourself can be extremely powerful, too. You're taking charge of your own well-being and, by extension, making sure that you remain available to others. Recognizing that we're all in this world together is a sign of emotional maturity. Indicating in clear and direct terms that you could do with a helping hand is not a sign of weakness. It's important to examine your ideas about asking for support. Nicci Gerrard is right when she states, "To be human is to be dependent; this isn't a weakness but a necessary condition of being alive. We are born helpless and we die helpless, and in between is the continual flux of giving and receiving, of being at each other's mercy, of helping others and of being helped in our turn."

How do you feel when you're able to help another person? Nine out of ten people answer this question with terms like "seen," "fulfilled," "social," "supportive," "relieved," "connected," and "valuable." We often don't stop to think that we may be doing somebody a favor by accepting help. Being open to support gives others a chance to feel helpful and useful and to gain new experiences.

Don't set the bar needlessly high. It's all right to ask for help with things you feel you could or should do on your own. The support you ask for also doesn't have to be practical. You could even say to a friend, "I need to get something off my chest; would you mind listening to me?" I'm always pleased when my father is very specific about his needs, whether it's buying new clothes for my mother or paying her an extra visit because he wants to do something else that day. Of course, my pleasure.

Giving help

If you don't need help yourself but you're not sure what you could do for someone else, why not ask a very direct question: "What's useful to you at this moment?" Not long ago, I heard from someone who'd kindly offered to go and get groceries, but it turns out that getting groceries was the primary caregiver's one opportunity to leave the house for a while. Instead, the helper spent an hour watching TV with the person with dementia, so his partner could stay out a bit longer. You'll work something out together.

Even when your offer of a helping hand isn't immediately accepted, be patient and continue to make yourself available. You could, for example, announce that in a week or two you'll come back and ask again. Stress that it's no effort, that you mean it, and that you're doing it out of respect and regard for the other. Another good strategy is to offer something very specific, like mowing the lawn or dropping off a home-made lasagna. The rejection of your support is more about a temporary prolonging of self-preservation and autonomy than it is about not wanting your help. Give it time.

Finally, the question "How are you doing?" is often too broad, too much. From now on, I suggest we ask each other, "How are you doing *right now*?"

DEMENTIA AND
MEANING

FINDING WORDS FOR WHAT CAN'T BE SAID

These days I don't always know how to get through to my mother, so we just stroll past the units of the home where she lives. The corridors form a square, so nobody gets lost. When we turn another corner, we come upon an old transistor radio. It's a so-called Snoezelen object, or multisensory object—something with lights and sounds to stimulate the senses of people with dementia. The radio emits static. I tap the cabinet and press a few buttons. Suddenly, the voice of Charles Aznavour fills the deserted corridor. "Shall we dance, Mom?" She raises her arms, I hold her in a tight embrace, and together we sway back and forth, while Aznavour sings: *She may be the mirror of my dream / a smile reflected in a stream.* Then the low afternoon sun pours in and bathes us in a brilliant light. A thousand little particles of dust dance around us. My mother gives me a kiss on the cheek and caresses my back, while I have tears rolling down my cheeks. It's such a fragile, magical moment. For a split second we simply "are," and that means everything to me. I'm dancing with my mother, heart to heart, bathed in the light of love and music. *Me, I'll take her laughter and her tears / and make them all my souvenirs.* "Thank you," I mutter, to no one in particular. I'm acutely aware of the importance of honoring, letting in moments of pure magic. I can't do without them.

They're like fireflies on the darkest days, enchanting little lights when everything's dull and gray. Let in magic and you let in the heart. Let in the heart and you let in the light.

When pain or grief crosses our path, we're really thrown for a loop. Everything we've taken for granted now feels unsteady and uncertain. It's at moments like these that major existential questions tend to germinate: What does it all mean? What are human beings and what's our purpose? What's the meaning of life? Maybe this is something you recognize. Faced with my mother's diagnosis and all the emotions it stirred, a very specific question came to my mind: Why has dementia crossed my path?

I've often wondered these past few years, as I've held my mother's hands in mine. I don't subscribe to the school of thought that believes that illnesses or other misfortunes come your way because you've got "something to learn" in this life—adversity with a *purpose*. To my mind that's an unnecessarily cruel, superficial interpretation of the pain and suffering in the world and in our lives. But I do believe that setbacks and grief, *if and when* they occur, bring an opportunity for learning. They can imbue the seemingly meaningless with meaning. So the question I now consider is, *How can I find meaning in dementia now that this illness has crossed my path?*

I'm not unique in the search for purpose and meaning. It's a quintessential part of being human. For me, it's also a coping mechanism. I'm always curious to see where other people turn to find courage, comfort, and resilience and where I might discover them for myself. There are times when the more challenging aspects of my mother's dementia make me sad and defiant. What's this good for? (Nothing.) Why do people have to go through this? (For no good reason.) Why my mother? (Why not her?) I draw on language and the imagination to make sense of the inner ping-pong between questions and answers about meaning. My father once messaged me something he'd heard on the radio: "Shadow is not the opposite of light; it's proof that there is light." That's a beautiful thought. Life embodies that duality: ebb and flow, day and night, temporal and eternal, yin and yang—they're not at odds with one another but instead complementary. The rough edges of life also show us what's valuable. Grief shows us what matters, what brings us meaning and happiness. Delving into the various religious, philosophical, and spiritual approaches to dementia is my way of finding a balance. It makes it possible for the meaninglessness of dementia to be offset by meaning, and that's comforting.

Health care professionals refer to the ideology that someone draws on to handle adversity as the "framework of meaning." The tools made available by such a framework can help you find comfort and reassurance. Psychologists are divided on whether spirituality constitutes a coping mechanism in and of itself, but the way we act and react based on a particular worldview certainly does. It influences the way we approach life and serves as a foundation for (self-) belief and surrender. "Trusting" and "having faith" give hope and strength—that's something numerous scholars agree on.

Spirituality not only contributes to resilience; it's an essential component of it, according to Brené Brown. In her book *Rising Strong*, she sets out the "rules" that help us come back stronger from adversity. Brown calls them the physics of vulnerability. One of the rules posits that rising strong is a spiritual exercise. After ten years of research, she reached the following conclusion: "Spirituality is recognizing and celebrating that we are all inextricably connected to one another by a power greater than all of us, and that our connection to that power and to one another is grounded in love and belonging. Practicing spirituality brings a sense of perspective, meaning, and purpose to our lives."

Are we talking about God? No idea. You could give what Brown describes as "a force greater than ourselves" a name that feels right to you. There are so many words for it: goodness, love, the divine, God, the light, the universe, the All. I often refer to it as "the source of life," inspired by the first line of the Lord's Prayer, as adapted by Bram Moerland. The original Aramaic is often translated as "Oh Thou, from whom the breath of life comes."

THE IMPORTANCE OF STORIES

The search for meaning is a natural part of being human. It doesn't have to come under the banner of religion. Sharing stories about love and suffering and darkness and light is as old as humanity itself and takes many forms. From myths passed down orally to contemporary fairytales, from sacred texts to spiritual fables, they all seek to tell us something about the eternal dance of good and evil.

This longing for explanation is timeless and universal. The common thread in these stories is that suffering rarely "is what it is." More often than not, protagonists have to face challenges on their path before they can come out the other end and achieve peace, light, love, or another form of victory. Whether we're talking about Little Red Riding Hood or Jesus, Harry Potter or the Buddha, they're all pushed to the brink before they find redemption. Their trials and tribulations should help us trust that adversity doesn't necessarily spell the end but instead often holds the promise of a new beginning.

Issues of meaning and purpose are all about the road we have to travel. Stories help us to gain a better understanding of life. By putting ourselves in other people's shoes, we can safely experience what it means to be afraid yet show courage, to lose yet be triumphant. Identification with a story activates the same parts of the brain that the actual experience would have fired. The imagination enables us to be genuinely freaked out or have butterflies in our stomach. That means that when we have our own brush with misfortune, our imaginative powers and empathy will have given us some practice and resilience.

SUFFERING

Suffering is unavoidable. However much money you have in the bank, however hard you work, however many leafy green vegetables you eat, nobody is guaranteed a carefree life. The passing of time, illness, decline, goodbyes, and the grief this all causes—there's no averting or escaping any of it. To suffer is to be human, you might say. Dementia really rubs our noses in it: The illness not only causes you to watch your loved one suffer but also brings its own suffering to the beholder. When your loved one has a certain type of dementia or they're at an advanced stage, you'll be even more aware of the suffering than they are.

To bear this suffering, we must first understand something important: the distinction between being in pain and suffering. Pain is the objective presence of pure, physical discomfort or visceral emotions. It's pain we can't escape and a direct response to what's happening. Suffering comes next. It follows when we attach thoughts to what we're feeling and feelings to what we're thinking.

In essence, we suffer when we find ourselves in a situation that doesn't correspond to what we'd like reality to be.

Thupten Jinpa, whose book *A Fearless Heart* I mentioned earlier, writes, "Suffering is an inescapable part of our reality and the sooner we can develop a healthy relationship to it the better off we will be. The first step is to learn how to be with our own *pain and suffering*, without resistance and *without giving in* to the urge to find an immediate solution."

The distinction between pain and suffering cracks open the door to meaning. If they're not the same, it may be possible for suffering to be cathartic. That's no small thing. It's what I mean when I say that grief and pain can help us grow. You're always learning, not just when you're happy but also when you're suffering. You may not recognize it until years later, but there's a chance you'll discover something about yourself or about life. In that sense, suffering is a kind of learning path that sends us deep down into our heart. We go deep, yet live to tell the tale, recognizing that everything we want to cling to is ephemeral, imperfect, and always in flux. Since we have no choice, faced with dementia, we might as well let some seeds germinate in that profound darkness so they can grow toward the light. As the Dutch writer Susan Smit once said to me, "Enriching and deepening your experiences may well be the most important things that spirituality can do for you."

Kristin Neff's book *Self-Compassion* features a beautiful story from the Native American tradition. An old Cherokee man, eager to teach his grandson about life, explains to the boy that he has two wolves fighting inside of him: One is evil (representing anger, envy, sorrow, regret, and more difficult emotions) and the other is good (symbolizing peace, love, joy, hope, and the like). All people have such wolves fighting within, he tells his grandson, to which the boy asks, "Which wolf is going to win?" The man answers, "The wolf you feed."

SPIRITUAL BYPASSING

Perhaps at this point neither "meaning" nor "the bigger picture" is of any use to you. It's not my intention to cause irritation or resentment. Talking about dementia, especially dementia and meaning, is always going to be fraught. There's a lot going on with this illness, some of it intense and painful. When my mother is going through a difficult patch, I don't want to hear about "meaning" either. Sometimes it's just not the right time. If you're currently walking a steep section of the learning path with your loved one, then feel free to skip this chapter for now. Unfortunately, people with dementia don't spend their days sitting peacefully in a rocking chair with a blanket over their legs, singing songs from their childhood. My mother certainly isn't quite so serene; she's often sad, restless, or very withdrawn. Other residents in her nursing home find themselves in the same heart-rending situation. If meaning eludes you right now, you'll need to start by bringing all your attention to what's being asked of you.

It takes time and silence to explore and find meaning. And there's always a risk of *spiritual bypassing*, that is to say, the use of spirituality as a filter on reality. No longer a powerful and meaningful part of your approach to dementia, the search for meaning has turned into a kind of Bubble Wrap, designed to protect you from reality as it is. Spirituality can be an escape, a way of losing yourself in an alternative scenario in which there's no pain and grief and everything is just fine. But meaning without space for painful feelings is denial. In extreme cases, people even use spirituality to relieve themselves of the responsibility to be present in the here and now. Trust the process, they'll say, or some other snappy slogan, and that's supposed to be the end of the matter. Unfortunately, it doesn't work that way. Not everything difficult can be sidestepped with radical idealism. At best, it's been temporarily banished to your subconscious, where it continues to simmer. Ultimately, spiritual bypassing achieves the opposite of what spirituality can help you with: to be mindfully and compassionately present.

LEARNING TO TRUST

I view spirituality and meaning the same way I look at art or listen to music. To me, they're an interpretation of reality. All these different takes on life are poignant human efforts to explain the inexplicable and to bear the unbearable. What matters is not whether something is true but whether it's valuable to you and your loved one at this moment in time. Meaningful imagination lends color and depth to life. And while it may not change reality as it is, it does alter the backdrop against which we live our lives.

Following a spiritual path, any path, is all about learning to trust. Trusting that even the darkest night will eventually turn into morning. It's believing that life itself carries that promise, that pain will always be offset by pleasure, that light will follow dark—however unlikely it may seem right now.

This confidence can be a lifeline in the most turbulent waters. At times when my mother's dementia is troubling me most, when reality is undeniably raw, spirituality is a source of renewed focus and drive. It motivates me to act on what's valuable to me. It makes meaning more than just a nice story, something that really permeates the roots of life. Faced with dementia, it inspires us to look deep inside and to bring our love and soul to everything we do.

In an interview on a Dutch talk show, Hans Korteweg, a writer, teacher, and master in the art of living, spoke beautifully about his wife's dementia. His words captured the essence what I feel.

> When someone's suffering from a serious illness, I'm wary of describing it as meaningful. I steer clear of any positive interpretation as an outsider. I can now say that what has happened to me, to my dear wife Hanneke,

over the past ten years . . . has been a blessing. But a
blessing that has put me through the wringer. It has also
brought profound sorrow. I have felt intensely isolated
and alone, but at the same time this has allowed me to
realize something I'd known all along. But what I knew
has gone from mere knowledge to something made flesh.
Instead of being enlightened, I want to serve. . . . What I
know about life, I now express through living.

A sense of meaning provides an incentive to get up in the morning, to want to keep trying for yourself and your loved one with dementia. No, spirituality isn't a miracle cure that takes away all the pain, sorrow, and adversity. Anyone who suggests otherwise is a charlatan. But almost all forms of spiritual, religious, or philosophical practice ultimately boil down to this: *staying with what is*, wanting to act from trust and love.

At a time when it's widely believed that we can create, solve, control, and explain everything, the mystical has been relegated to the sidelines. Our natural propensity for mysticism and the questions in our heart have been suppressed by the conviction that life can be shaped to meet our needs. There *has* to be a reason things are the way they are and, if at all possible, a solution, too. Some will therefore dismiss an interest in meaning and purpose as an escape from reality. But I think the opposite is true—embracing and exploring the unfamiliar and the undefined will allow you to experience reality more intensely.

A SENSE OF MEANING
PROVIDES AN INCENTIVE TO
GET UP IN THE MORNING, TO
WANT TO KEEP TRYING FOR
YOURSELF AND YOUR LOVED
ONE WITH DEMENTIA.

And why not? Having one's head in the clouds is a welcome alternative to the dementia grinding us down. There are many approaches to thinking spiritually about dementia, ranging from an esoteric take on consciousness to the perspective of a Christian God. What if somewhere else my mother's incoherent sounds constitute a language that *does* make sense? What if the long-drawn-out conclusion to her life here is a gentle beginning elsewhere? Merely allowing myself these thoughts gives me the headspace to view my mother and her illness in a different, better, and softer light.

A COSMIC CONSCIOUSNESS

You may have noticed that a dementia patient can look absent, somewhere far beyond the horizon, invisible and inaccessible to others. By the same token, my mother's eyes can be unfathomably calm and deep. At those moments her gaze reminds me of that of a newborn baby: wise and tranquil.

Spiritual movements often speak of a "cosmic consciousness," or different layers of consciousness. Our subconscious taps into this boundless, infinite source of wisdom and love, where all is good and safe. We are born of this cosmic consciousness, as reflected in an infant's gaze, and it's what we return to, according to the spiritual teachers in these circles. Our thinking mind, consciousness, and our perception of reality act as a kind of filter between this cosmic network and day-to-day life. This is necessary, because we must weigh and work with all the information we receive during our earthly existence. However, as beliefs and patterns become more entrenched over time, that filter between the subconscious and the conscious becomes more rigid and opaque. So the more you can open up, the more easily you can move through the layers of consciousness.

Spiritual experiences, those instances when you feel at one with everything and in harmony with the cosmos, are the moments when you've found or created an opening in that filter. That's why babies look so wise to us—the filter has barely been formed. The pure, cosmic energy between the conscious and subconscious can flow freely. When you view dementia through that lens, the illness can create a gateway to this cosmic consciousness where there's no time, no judgment, and no pain. As the filter of consciousness is dissolved, someone with dementia travels between the dimensions, which is why sometimes they're alert and present and sometimes far away in unfathomable depths.

A subset within this way of looking at the world believes that people with dementia can free themselves from whatever keeps them tied to this earthly life. By casting off the mental shackles while we're still alive, the soul becomes light and pure. It allows someone with the illness to discard all worldly baggage and, free from suffering, return to the cosmic consciousness as a pure, enlightened soul. Some people feel this speaks to them, others not at all, and that's fine.

You will know what best fits your personal experience and framework of meaning.

THE SPIRIT OF NATURE

The natural world doesn't occupy a prominent place in our framework of meaning. In fact, a connection with nature seems less of a given these days, as if it's something separate from us. Our top priorities are to grow as old as possible, to remain strong and active for as long as possible, and to wither as little as possible. So we apply expensive anti-wrinkle creams, supermarkets sell only unblemished fruit, and when we want to know what the weather is like we look not outside but at our phones. The natural world is supposed to serve us, and we place ourselves above and beyond it.

Yet here in the West we've certainly had a tradition of old nature religions in which the power of the natural world takes center stage, like it did in ancient Celtic and Germanic cultures. In other parts of the world, like South America, such faiths remain more widely practiced. These nature religions have a very different understanding of the natural phenomena and processes around us than most of us are used to. One belief they all share is that every element of creation has a spirit and that the cycle of life is the eternal source from which everything springs and to which everything returns. Just like the sun rises and sets, the moon waxes and wanes, plants and flowers bloom and wilt, and humans and animals are born and die. None of these processes happen independently of us; we're part of them. That's why we must respect nature, the giver and taker of life, and honor and nurture our relationship with it.

The "self" doesn't play a dominant, leading role in nature religions. Everything begins and ends with nature. The natural world is intricate, complex, and vast, and as individuals we're insignificant cogs in this machine. This is incompatible with the whole idea of human beings as somehow separate from creation. The dementia of a loved one also takes on a new meaning in this light: Somebody is and always will be part of an ever-changing creation. The spirit, or what you might call the "soul" or the inner "life force," is present in everything around us. While we tend to see the process of dementia as someone's gradual disappearance, their spirit is never actually gone. It's reabsorbed in the greater consciousness of everything in existence. The "self" isn't limited or finite. The spirit is found in a flower in bloom, in a fluttering butterfly, a rainstorm, or a rock formation.

Nature religions respect what's known as "cyclical time." Think of the tides, the circadian rhythms, and the recurring seasons. Time is perceived not just as a linear path from A to B but as a circle. Everything in nature keeps going back to the beginning in a perpetual cycle. Germinating, growing, flowering, and withering, over and over. When I went with a friend to visit her mother in a nursing home, the mother said to us, "I have this sense that my mom is still alive." She was referring to my friend's grandmother and she was still lucid enough to know that this wasn't the case, yet the feeling was very strong—as if she were going back to the beginning. My own mother will sometimes quietly murmur "Mom," as though she's edging closer to where it all started for her.

Seeing life as cyclical, mindful of the natural rhythm of coming and going, can help us view death and disease with a more open mind. Mortality is a natural part of any life cycle. We're not sad when the trees drop their leaves in the fall and winter returns. If we apply this approach to dementia, we may become more accepting of the process.

SPEAKING OF GOD

In the Netherlands, many of the older generations are likely to situate their framework of meaning within the Judeo-Christian tradition, as it is historically most intertwined with Dutch culture. That being said, both in the Netherlands and elsewhere in the world, the Christian landscape is extremely varied. Ask five random people about their idea of God and you'll probably hear five different worldviews that have, as their source, the same deity. It will be difficult to distill any universal insight about dealing with dementia from this.

However liberal or orthodox your outlook may be, all Christian denominations share common ground. Mankind was created in God's image, for example, which means that all human beings are perfect and precious, regardless of medical history or social standing. As Martin Luther King Jr. used to say, all people are equal in the eyes of God. In fact, perhaps it's the most vulnerable who need our care the most. The stories about Jesus's life certainly seem to bear witness to this. The unconditional love of a heavenly father, as preached in Christianity, can be invaluable in dealing with dementia, as is the Christian concept of charity. These aren't just empty phrases, especially not when love can no longer be reciprocated and it's up to you to treat others the way you'd want to be treated yourself. "Doing God is doing good" is how a theologian friend of mine puts it. Whatever your take on God, we can all work on doing good.

While I was reading about the various Christian perspectives on dementia, I came across a text from the Gospel of Luke. In it, Jesus says, "Let the little children come to me, and do not hinder them, for the kingdom of God belongs to such as these" (New International Version, 18:16). It's a verse that's often quoted in relation to dementia. People with the illness are sometimes described as "childlike" because they no longer abide by the adult rules pertaining to self-sufficiency and social interaction. Does that mean that, from a Christian point of view, people with dementia are close to God or a heavenly paradise?

I put this thought to my theologian friend. "That's a view I share," he says. "In this text, the word 'child' stands not for naivety but for purity, helplessness, and vulnerability. Jesus is speaking in the course of a conversation with his disciples, who want to know who's the most eminent, the most important to him. His response: 'Let the children come to me, and do not hinder them, for the Kingdom of God belongs to such as these'" (Luke 18:16). My friend quotes another Bible text that he often thinks of while supporting people with dementia. It's Psalm 139: "O Lord, you have searched me and known me." This, too, is about our *essence*, the purity far beyond status and identity, which a person with dementia is forced to relinquish.

As I was exploring these Christian perspectives, I also came across a work by John Swinton, a Scottish theologian and professor. He has written a (rather dry) tome about his Christian perspective on dementia. The treatise is known within theological circles, but it's not really the kind of book that I, a layperson, can come to grips with. It's the title of Swinton's study that appeals to me—*Dementia: Living in the Memories of God*. What could it mean? What's the point of God remembering you when you can't remember yourself? Being in somebody's memories when your own memories are gone? In the Netherlands, "dementia pastor" Tim van Iersel addresses similar issues, including the question of whether it's possible to believe in God when you've forgotten who God is.

The comforting thought for me is that while a person can forget *themself*, that doesn't mean that they *are* forgotten. A relationship based on unconditional love transcends both the thinking mind and linear time and encapsulates a time-less, divine essence. I can't resist placing this idea in a larger framework of meaning, because I think it's beautiful and not just within a strictly Christian context. What if we replace God with "the divine" or "the source of life" or another term that you feel comfortable with? What if we let the person we love so much live on in our memories?

For Swinton, remembering isn't just literal recollection but also *re-membering*, constantly reconnecting with people. It's about bringing people back into the fold, again and again, making sure they remain in our lives and in our hearts. When my mother no longer recognizes me, no longer calls me by my name, and even forgets that she loves me, I keep reconnecting and remembering (on her behalf) and she will be affirmed, seen, and known. In this way we carry everybody with dementia in our hearts, collectively, for as long as we can, and nobody is ever forgotten. Those who are remembered never die.

WHAT DOES MY MOTHER THINK?

Of course I'm curious to know what kind of meaning my mother would have given to the dementia that crossed her path. She approached life in a very liberal Protestant way. She didn't believe in the traditional God up in heaven but did place herself within the Judeo-Christian tradition. The extraordinary thing is that I'm not *completely* in the dark about her views. When my mother was in her forties and my brothers and I were somewhat older, she started a theology degree to become a pastoral worker. In 1994, she wrote her undergraduate thesis. Titled *Woorden ten leven*, or "Words for Life," it looked at the role of language and metaphor in pastoral work with women "finding their voice." The essay had a feminist slant and challenged the religious patriarchy. My mother looked specifically at instances of misogynist language within the church tradition, with God the Almighty Father as the Supreme Being.

It really saddens me that I never had any profound conversations with her about religion and meaning—at the time of her degree I was still too young to be interested. These themes have now become the focus of my own work: comfort, courage, and resilience, and how and where to find them. They're at the heart of what I write for *Happinez* magazine and in my books. I think she's proud of that. In her own thesis, which I frequently dip into, my mother writes, "Language is a vital tool for expressing how we see ourselves and the world." It's almost as if she left a time capsule with words so that I could find encouragement and solace on my path. She also states, "We become human through language." How painful to think that language was one of the first things she was robbed of by the dementia.

I read between the lines of her thesis to discover what might bring her comfort now and stumble upon a passage in which she writes about the importance of listening. In spiritual support work, she argues, when you're listening to the other person's story, you're doing it as much on your own as on God's behalf. If you're really there for somebody else, you are more than just a listener, a vehicle for the divine, the good. As she notes, "Every meaningful relationship between people has a dimension that transcends the relationship itself." This fits in very nicely with the search for meaning and dementia, because the care relationship has such a transcendent element, too. It's *being* together. I sincerely hope that my mother feels the same, that the divine, the good, is always there with and between us. That's certainly my experience.

ABOUT THE SELF

"Remember, you're not your thoughts," the yoga instructor says during a class. I smile and, thinking of my mother, switch it around: My mom no longer thinks about herself. It's an extraordinary paradox: We're very attached to our thinking mind and our autonomy, and yet much of our spiritual practice is aimed at freeing us from the "self." Moments when we're able to slow our raging torrent of thoughts to a calm, babbling brook are often described as "spiritual awakening." When we identify the pause button of the mind and we can simply *be* in the moment, we speak of "becoming one with the universe" or of "enlightenment"—for many the ultimate spiritual ideal. We want to get out of our head, but at the same time dementia, the true liberation from the thinking mind, is our greatest fear. Where does dementia leave the "self"?

Dementia does away with the thinking mind's dominant role when we're not even trying, let alone asking, for it. Those with a radical spiritual take on dementia view their loved one's illness as a form of enlightenment, describing it as a beautiful process of transformation and detachment from the self and the ego. For me, this interpretation goes too far, although it does raise some interesting ideas.

Being human is often encapsulated in the concepts of body, mind, and soul. Some use body, reason, and emotion; or else body, intellect, and heart—all of which boil down to more or less the same thing. Together these three elements form the essence of our humanity. The heart needs the thinking mind to arrive at informed decisions, and vice versa. In this process the body serves as a sounding board with whispered cues and screaming alarm bells: a beating heart, a lump in your throat, a stomach full of butterflies. In dementia, at least two of the three—the thinking mind and the body—are eroded by illness. When the thinking mind is no longer capable of expressing identity, it's said that that person "is no longer there." What does that mean? Who *are* we?

The Dutch author Hans Stolp argues that the impairment of the physical thinking mind makes it harder for the spirit (i.e., the soul) "to guide us in life." He writes, "It has no choice but to gradually withdraw, and to some extent leave the physical body." As Stolp sees it, this explains why people with dementia appear distant or have a vacant look in their eyes; as the soul withdraws from the physical body, its link with the spiritual world grows stronger. Where beholders mostly see progressive deterioration, an invisible process of healing and acceptance is taking place. The spiritual world is all love, and this is beneficial to the soul.

People with dementia certainly still experience a *self*, albeit one that no longer conforms to our expectations and memories. While I was researching this book, this was confirmed to me by doctors and caregivers who encounter it daily and act accordingly, for example, by always addressing the patient directly and with respect. The staff at my mother's nursing facility do this incredibly well—sometimes even better than I do—by never talking down to her and never losing sight of her autonomy. On the evening of my mother's first day there, I was carrying some of her possessions to her room when I overheard a conversation between the senior care worker and a colleague. They were drawing up her care plan but couldn't complete all the necessary forms. "Let's leave it for now and focus on getting to know her first," one said to the other. "We'll take our time to find out who she is and what she likes." Not only did they show great integrity and respect for my mother, but they also put my mind at ease. She was seen as a *person*.

"She's no longer there" is a very strange thing to say. You wouldn't describe a baby that can't make its own decisions, clearly express itself, or look after itself as somehow not a person. The difference is that our loved one is no longer the individual we once knew—and that's significant. Throughout life, our identity, our self, never stops developing and changing. We learn new things, form new opinions, and master new skills. We're like paintings that keep acquiring new accents—sometimes these are applied in thick splotches, sometimes in wafer-thin daubs of color. When do we think a change in identity or the disappearance of an earlier self has gone too far? Doesn't the malfunction of the thinking mind and the body leave a purer self? At times my mother may be hidden under thick layers of unusual behavior or extreme absent-mindedness, but she is still here.

That's why, among all the old photos stuck to the fridge, there's now a new one of my mother and me. She has her head on my chest and a smile on her lips. I look at the lens, but she's not aware of the camera at all. You can tell that she's ill. The dementia has been pictured, too. It makes me a bit sad, as she's not the mother I once knew. But she's the mother I have now, and I'm determined to love both her *and* her illness unconditionally and to give them a place in my life. It's up to me to honor her *self* in all its different guises. So, let's keep taking photos and capturing our loved ones on camera—they don't stop where the dementia begins.

Advice from a person with dementia

- The way you look at me and talk to me has a significant effect on how I feel.

- Sometimes I'm impatient, angry, or emotional because I don't understand everything that's happening. Don't take it personally.

- It may look as if I no longer hear or see everything, but I'm aware when you talk over my head.

- It takes a while for the meaning of words and phrases to sink in, so please be patient with me. Go slow, calm down, and be gentle when you're talking to me.

- My personal space is important to me. This is where I keep my possessions and memories and I get to be fully myself.

- Inside I'm still the person I used to be. I've been through a lot in my life and I carry my experiences and emotions with me.

People with dementia are incredibly intuitive. When your inner compass isn't clouded by thoughts about what you feel and by feelings about what you're thinking, your intuition can become clear. That's why people with dementia are often sensitive to external stimuli and the mood of those around them, just like small children. This has been found in scientific research, as Huub Buijssen wrote: "We now know that for a long time after the diagnosis, a person with dementia continues to possess a so-called theory of mind, the human capacity for imagining what another feels or thinks in a particular situation."

In its early stages, dementia mainly damages the outer layers of the brain. Emotions are located much deeper and often remain unaffected for some time. People with dementia still have feelings. In fact, they likely intensify when all else falls away. This explains why music or art therapy can be so beneficial: Intense emotions and experiences remain long after the thinking mind is impaired. Beyond the forest of fallen leaves is an interior garden where the roses are still in bloom.

My father is a great lover of music, a conductor, singer, and multi-instrumentalist. He listens to music with my mom, and the minute he sits down at the piano in her nursing home, he attracts a small crowd. Around Christmas, he and a few friends from his choir sing in my mother's home, and I'm moved to tears. People who are normally withdrawn and hardly ever speak are suddenly singing along to Christmas carols from their childhood or moving in time to the music with their eyes closed. In the Netherlands, the Muziek als Medicijn (Music as Medicine) foundation, which is affiliated with the Erasmus University Medical Center in Rotterdam, has done a lot of research into music in caregiving, including for dementia, and has put the subject on the map. The comfort and sense of belonging that an art form like music can provide resonates profoundly, far beyond reason or the thinking mind.

While the self may not always be immediately apparent, it's certainly present. Thinking about the self and identity in relation to dementia is complex and extremely emotional. It raises big questions about being human: Who and what are you when you have dementia? Since we place such value on the thinking mind when our brain is healthy, does that mean that our soul, or our essence, our *being* plays second fiddle to it?

My mother's social worker told me that in the past ten years the number of people raising the topic of euthanasia in her consulting room has skyrocketed. That's extraordinary. My own observations bear this out, as does media coverage. In 2021, a Dutch newspaper published an interview with the journalist Clairy Polak, who lost her husband to dementia. The headline of the piece was: "If I were diagnosed with Alzheimer's, I wouldn't hesitate to take my own life." That's heavy. Obviously, it's her decision, one that's informed by her own experiences with dementia. This predominantly negative perception of the illness, and categorical rejection, leaves in its wake all those who suffer from it. This lack of nuance doesn't make it any easier for anyone to arrive at a balanced decision, neither those who are diagnosed nor their nearest and dearest.

Language matters. How we talk about something is how we shape reality. If we can't get past descriptions like awful, dehumanizing, sad, and apocalyptic, then that's what dementia will be. It's only when we also find words for the gentler aspects of the disease that we can do the whole experience justice. Both the illness and the ill person deserve stories of encouragement and words of comfort.

People tend to be firm in their rejection of a future with dementia; the loss of autonomy and identity weigh heavy. It seems that you no longer amount to much as soon as you get dementia. "What saddens me is that the healthy 'self' rejects the ill 'self' out of hand," my mother's social worker said to me. "But we don't address the underlying reasons. Where does this fear come from and how realistic is it? What have you been taught about independence and dependence?"

We have become so obsessed with control and self-determination that we sometimes see having a self-described identity as the definition of being human. That said, I completely understand the desire for free choice, and I don't know what my mother would have wanted for herself if she'd had the chance to give it clear and sustained thought. But we need to move away from the idea that dementia is nothing but suffering if we genuinely want to arrive at well-considered judgments on behalf of our loved one. We often fail to see the whole picture.

In most cases, it never comes to assisted suicide, because people in the throes of dementia often forget they even thought about it and do experience some quality of life. And that's in conflict with two of the key conditions for euthanasia: a considered request and unbearable suffering. When assisted suicide is something you and your loved one might consider, you'll have to talk about it at the earliest possible opportunity, and this conversation will have to be carefully documented. But most people miss the boat before they even get to that stage. That's why it's so important to meet dementia with an open mind, without prejudice, and look at it from all possible angles. You simply have no other choice.

WHY?

Why did my mother get ill? Why was our family struck by dementia? Why do I have to miss my mother while she's still alive? Why am I forced to deal with the reckoning this illness brings? I'm sure you recognize these questions; sooner or later we all ask them, often against our better judgment, because we know we won't get conclusive answers. "Why?" is an existential question that has its roots in human suffering. Even Jesus asked it on the cross: "My God, my God, why have you forsaken me?"

The purest, most honest answer is that dementia is a progressive, incurable disease that can affect any of us, because we have a body that can and will break down eventually, however sad that may be. Sometimes that answer will suffice, sometimes it won't—at vulnerable moments, especially, the "why" question keeps rearing its intrusive head.

I've taken a radical approach as far as the "why" question is concerned: I no longer pay attention to it because it won't help me in the long run. The thinking mind can come up with a thousand different answers, likely with big dollops of guilt and a generous serving of "what-ifs," but eventually they're all undone by the reality of what is.

If we want to interrogate fate in our efforts to deal with dementia, we'd better learn to ask different questions. I certainly derive courage and strength from replacing the intimidating word "why" with the more enabling and productive "how." "Why" forces you to think about the past and the things we can't change, but "how" can give us a new perspective. It shifts your attention to the future, to opportunities and solutions. "How" sparks a different kind of thought process, one with room for creativity, hope, and resilience: How can I learn to handle everything that my mother's dementia throws at me?

Edith Eger, a writer and Holocaust survivor, captures this dilemma well. Instead of "why," she asks herself, "What next?" One of my favorite books, *Tiny Beautiful Things* by Cheryl Strayed, has a dog-eared page that reads: "So here's the long and short of it [. . .]: there is no why. You don't have a right to the cards you believe you should have been dealt. You have an obligation to play the hell out of the ones you're holding."

Is there such a thing as "fate"? I'm afraid there's no clear answer to that either. Does everything just happen to us, or is it predestined? Do we have any influence over our lives? Some neuroscientists claim that there's no free will because our brain has already decided all our actions, reactions, and choices for us. Our path through life is thought to be largely shaped by a cocktail of the past, circumstance, and genetic traits—the principle of determinism in a nutshell. Various spiritual and religious movements see things differently. In Hinduism, for example, the course of your current life is said to be the outcome of what you did in your previous one. Others, including people with an Islamic or Christian background, will say that God has a plan for you, which prompts the counterargument that humankind has also been created with free will. Then there are those who are adamant that you're in charge of your own destiny, as long as you go about manifesting your wishes and desires in the right way.

Walking the middle way (as the Buddha would advise) means accepting that you have some influence over your life, but that you should also surrender to whatever crosses your path. We're not puppets of the strings of fate, nor are we totally at the mercy of chance. We make decisions, big and small, every day: We get out of bed or not, we seek help or not. Taken together, all these actions have an effect, as this quote, which is sometimes attributed to Lao-tzu, suggests: "Watch your thoughts; they become words. Watch your words; they become actions. Watch your actions; they become habits. Watch your habits; they become character. Watch your character; it becomes your destiny."

Whether or not that destiny comes with a predetermined purpose we'll never really know. The question of why my mother has dementia always brings me back to the belief I shared at the start of this book: I don't think dementia happens for a specific reason, but when it crosses your path, you can find meaning in it. That's the difference between "why" and "how."

Destiny or not, it's understandable that now and then you feel extremely sad or angry about what has befallen you, regardless of your framework of meaning. Fate feels highly personal when it is actually impersonal. The fact that the natural world is ultimately indifferent is hard to accept. Life is tough and painful, not because we've done anything wrong or deserve suffering but because nature and all that lives and breathes in it are equal before the eyes of the cosmos.

Megan Devine wrote a book about grief, *It's OK That You're Not OK*, in which I came across these precious words that explain it well: "Grief is not an enlightenment program for a select few. No one needs intense, life-changing loss to become who they are 'meant' to be. The universe is not causal in that way; you need to become something, so life gives you this horrible experience in order to make it happen. On the contrary: Life is call-and-response. Things happen, and we absorb and adapt. We respond to what we experience, and that is neither good nor bad. It simply is. The path forward is integration, not betterment."

The thing about dementia, or any other illness or twist of fate, is this: Your plans or desires don't really come into it. We have no choice but to put up with the vagaries of life, which come with the territory. At best, we can make small tweaks or adjustments. As the philosopher Kierkegaard put it: "Life is not a problem to be solved but a reality to be experienced." Thankfully, having the courage to admit questions is what makes life special; it inspires us to discover, explore, travel, read, listen, watch, marvel, and imagine.

I won't entertain the notion that somebody may have dementia "for a reason" or has somehow "brought it on themselves." In the West the principle of karma is such an overworked concept, so divorced from its original meaning. For many people it means "What goes around comes around," but that's not really what it is. *Karma* is Sanskrit for "action" or "deed," and in its most basic sense it refers to the universal law of action and reaction. If you throw a rock into the water, the surface will ripple. Every action has consequences. But there's no hidden agenda: no judgment, no punishment, and no reward either.

The idea that a person might develop dementia for a reason, "because of karma," can set a toxic thought process in motion. It leads you down a path of crime and punishment, a dark road without space for comforting insights. If you want to give karma a place in your life, then let it flow from within. Act with loving-kindness and patience in the knowledge that sooner or later you'll reap the rewards. You have little or no influence over external factors, but what you do here and now is your choice and an opportunity for you to open your heart.

BEING WITH
"WHAT IS"

TOWARD MORE RESILIENCE AND ACCEPTANCE

Have you heard of *via ferrata*? Literally "iron path," it's a climbing route with steel cables or metal rungs fixed to the side of a mountain. Every few feet you reattach yourself and progress a bit farther. Should you fall, you'll still be dangling from the cable. It allows people without highly advanced climbing skills to safely negotiate sheer, inaccessible slopes. What's that got to do with dementia, you ask. A via ferrata is a good metaphor for the process of acceptance that's required of you in the face of this illness. Acceptance is the steel cable affixed to the steep mountain that you secure yourself to every few steps so as not to plunge into the depths.

The nature of dementia forces us to break acceptance down into a great many small steps. Acceptance involves resting and resigning. With dementia this has to be done gradually and repeatedly, every time a new normal is established and every time there's another setback or loss along the way. "I wish every visit could be the same as the one before," my father says, because the unpredictability is so unsettling. No sooner do we get our footing than the trapdoor opens and we have to regain our balance. What acceptance can do for us, in concrete terms, is to help us feel secure in the moment, in the here and now.

THE FIRST STEP IN THE

PROCESS OF ACCEPTANCE

WILL ALWAYS BE TO FEEL

WHAT YOU'RE FEELING.

Accepting a situation is easier said than done. At its most basic level it's the art of recognizing a situation for what it is. It's saying "yes" to the dementia as it unfolds and not resisting it. Strangely enough, accepting pain in the moment is the way of least pain. You can feel this in your body by exhaling and releasing the tension: Your shoulders will physically drop half an inch. Not accepting it will result in cramping, both physically and emotionally, and consume a lot of energy.

As I described in the chapter on challenges, the dementia of your loved one will stir up all kinds of emotions, including anger, denial, sadness—they're all part of the process. As a result, there's plenty for you to accept, from little everyday things that weren't a problem before to fundamental changes like nursing home admission or another medical setback. Let it be clear, you may not be able to respond with immediate acceptance. Often, you must first feel your way around challenges. This is an honest and pure reaction. If anything, clinging to your resistance will be your undoing in the end. Constantly fighting reality causes detachment at a moment when you really need to bring all your attention, love, and energy to the situation.

The first step in the process of acceptance will always be to feel what you're feeling. Emotions can wash over you like a big, powerful wave. When that happens, it's essential to keep treading water. "Feel your feelings" is good advice: Before you direct your attention to anything else, sit down with them. Feel what must be felt, without judgment, while being present in your body. Emotion is energy in motion. It comes and goes; it ebbs and flows.

The second stage involves your thinking mind. Take a step back and ask yourself: What's happening here? Do I understand what I'm seeing? These are important questions. Knowledge about dementia helps, as does sharing experiences and feelings with people who are also close to your loved one or who also have someone in their life with dementia. They may be able to come up with fresh insight, a different perspective, or words of comfort. Zooming out is always a good alternative to acting and reacting straight from your emotions; it may help you to arrive at a different, better solution or a new understanding.

Revising your expectations will often leave you better prepared for any plot twists. That way, any uncertainty about the latest manifestation of the disease is less likely to come as a major shock or disappointment to you. During the current stage of my mother's illness, for example, she keeps having minor seizures that are not uncommon in dementia. Knowing that they're part of the process makes them no less unpleasant, but at least we're not caught completely unawares, and we're not totally destabilized by each piece of bad news about her health. Acceptance softens the blow.

The third step is learning to surrender. The moments when you're able to surrender to the situation, without drowning in resistance and emotion, are the moments when you're left with more energy and clarity for the things you *can* control.

Acceptance is not about becoming passive or resigned but about drawing on your inner calm and loyalty to find the strength to keep moving forward. The emotions and challenges will still be there, but they no longer limit you in your endeavors in the here and now: being present, giving love, providing care. It's a major lesson in humility. It reminds me of a line by Cheryl Strayed: "Accept that this experience taught you something you didn't want to know."

It will not always be possible to muster that inner acceptance at every stage of the illness, and that's all right. Acceptance is never "complete," but always a work in progress. We're skaters, tracing infinite loops of acceptance and sadness on the ice. I see this in my father; every time my mother deteriorates, he has to readjust and go through the whole figure eight again. And again and again and again. The present moment is always temporary and unpredictable in dementia; the situation as it is *now* and what's acceptable *now* can be very different tomorrow and send you back into that loop.

Finally, acceptance isn't always about the big leaps in physical or mental decline. Mundane things also require us to let go of resistance, judgment, or desires. My mother has started grinding her teeth, louder than frogs croaking their mating call beside a pond. It's a deafening, irritating noise that raises eyebrows. I can't say: Stop it! While this may work briefly, in the end it's an involuntary tic and my resistance to it is pointless.

Practicing acceptance is also about the small stuff. While my mother's hair is nicely washed and cut, it's not styled the way she used to do herself. Sometimes the caregivers will give her a necklace to wear that doesn't go with her sweater. Her room has linoleum flooring in an indeterminate shade of lilac, whereas my mom loves bright colors. I've taken to buying her non-wired bras that are more comfortable when you're sitting down for much of the day. Who cares? Acceptance, acceptance, acceptance. The question I keep asking is, Does it really matter? Do I want my mother and her life to conform to what *I* think is nice and "normal"? Do I want to cover up all signs of her dementia, because *I* can't accept the advancing illness? Or do I want her to be surrounded by love, attention, and safety? It's the latter I want. It's not always straightforward to let go and ease up—in fact, it's often very hard—but everything that's a distraction from what really matters will become easier with acceptance.

Some of the things we must accept

- However patiently you explain something, the other person doesn't understand.
- Your loved one recoils from your touch.
- They lack initiative to carry out routine activities.
- They have no interest in things you care about, like your children, hobbies, or job.
- Past hurt is forgotten, but so are your fun and cherished memories together.

- Things are lost, both insignificant items and objects that you value.
- Unjustified accusations are leveled at you.
- Sudden mood swings will happen without any apparent reason.
- You're unable to comfort the other person in their anger or sadness.
- They lie and fabricate all the time.
- You receive no reaction to anything you say or do.
- You can no longer physically handle the other person and they don't cooperate.
- Their appearance and posture are completely different from before.
- Nothing you do can take away their suspicion and panic.
- Their tics, like fidgeting and pacing, make you nervous.
- You're left with little time to yourself, as they are very clingy.
- They see things or people that aren't there.
- Your expectations about each day go up in smoke.
- What you think is "normal" is no longer the norm.
- You no longer have a relationship of equals.
- Someone else suddenly becomes the "favorite" or is given a role that used to be yours.
- Questions, stories, or actions are endlessly repeated.

FORGIVENESS

When a person's rational and emotional capacities are impaired due to dementia, which affects the brain, you can no longer have a proper conversation with them. It's especially difficult when there are topics you would have wanted to discuss, but now can't. In any relationship, some conversations are delayed. "We'll get around to it later," we think, or "Now's not the right time." But when dementia comes into play, "not now" turns into "not ever." Everything you want to say about difficult moments between you and your loved one is shelved indefinitely. Or maybe nothing's been left unsaid between the two of you, but you just want them to explain something.

Perhaps deep down you long for forgiveness for the way that you initially dealt with the incipient dementia, for not saying "sorry," or for not expressing sooner how much you love them. When a relationship changes, and one person becomes dependent on the other, an entirely new dynamic emerges in which vulnerability comes to the fore.

I'm no stranger to wanting forgiveness. I'd love to ask my mother to forgive me. In the early stages of her illness, she was unable to budge an inch, thereby robbing us of the ability to provide better care. *Mom, I get it now.* To my father, who kept glossing over any ugliness, I want to say, *Dad, I understand.* Then there's me, who has to live with the question of whether we did the right thing or if we did *enough.* And, having cursed it, I'd like to ask forgiveness of the dementia itself. Pain and guilt are heavy burdens to bear and can prevent you from being present with attention and love. In that sense, forgiveness offers a way out of the labyrinth of regret, old hurt, and unresolved issues. Maybe you're familiar with this expression: "Forgiveness means giving up all hope for a better past."

We often think of forgiveness as an exchange, as something we give or receive from another person—a box filled with apology and regret. Dementia gets in the way of that dynamic. There's no chance of an exchange, acknowledgment, or regret, let alone hope of improvement or a different future. You'll have to find your own way out of the labyrinth. But you can take comfort from this: Forgiveness has always been a one-person project. Genuine forgiveness isn't something that's handed to you; it has to come from within. The only person who can deliver you from guilt, shame, and sadness is you.

Arriving at a place of forgiveness isn't easy. It's an internal process that calls for focus and commitment. This may explain why it has such an elevated position in many religions and forms of spirituality, and reinforces the idea that forgiveness requires an almost superhuman effort and is the reserve of gods and gurus. But we should rethink this idea of forgiveness as something imposed from above or beyond us and bring it back to human dimensions. I encourage you to stand in front of the mirror and to really feel that we're all trudging through the same earthly mud; that none of us is without faults or without flaws. We often inadvertently hurt or upset one another, because we're clumsy, weak, and sometimes just plain stupid. This is our common humanity. And in the face of something as unfamiliar and incomprehensible as dementia, it's no great sin when things don't go according to plan.

On the path that you and I walk together as we deal with dementia there's so much that's not under our control. And that's the beauty of forgiveness: It's something that we *do* have some influence over. Here lies an opportunity to make a difference. We can cut the strings that tie us to the past and enable everybody involved to proceed with less baggage. We have an opportunity to free both ourselves and the other person from old hurt, even if reciprocity is no longer an option.

Forgiving doesn't equal justifying or forgetting. It's acknowledging what is, feeling the emotional charge that comes with it, and yet actively choosing to move toward the light. This calls for empathy, honesty, patience, courage, and willpower, but it can be done. Forgiveness, every little bit of it, is a balm for the heart and soul, smoothing over scars and rough edges, because it stops the past from getting in the way of a cherished present. The time you have left with your loved one is simply too precious for that to happen. Having the space for kindness and tenderness will feed into all aspects of your life, including the way you handle dementia.

LIVING IN THE PRESENT

I genuinely think that living in the present is one of the greatest aspirations of our time. We live in a world full of frantic activity, stimuli, obligations, worries, and ambitions. Trying to escape it all has become big business. More and more people are practicing mindfulness and meditation, seeking peace of mind by traveling to far-flung places, attending expensive workshops, or heading out into nature to try and slow down. Leisure is the new gold. We'll do anything for a bit of peace amid the noise.

Wanting to be present is an admirable goal. The ability to free yourself from agonizing over the past and worrying about the future brings inner peace and calm. Those moments when I lose track of time and am fully absorbed in the now are my favorites. No obligations, not feeling like I have to juggle a thousand things. You briefly feel as if you get to ride in the passenger seat of life, leaning back and enjoying the view instead of keeping your eyes fixed on the road ahead.

Our thinking mind isn't necessarily wired to live in the moment. We look back and look ahead as a survival strategy. Everything we experience is stored in our memory, so we can react quickly and adequately to new events. Burn yourself once and you'll keep away from the flames in the future. However, the more experiences accumulate and translate into convictions, habits, and patterns, the harder it becomes to be in the moment. That's why, for many people, living in the now is as much exertion as it is relaxation—it's difficult to disengage from the chokehold of everyday life, the maelstrom of thoughts and the feelings they evoke.

Why are we so eager to be present? Because it creates peace and quiet, in your head as well as in your body. In both spiritual and scientific circles people who are "mentally flexible"—that's to say, those who have developed the ability to create space or a pause between thinking and being—are known to experience greater calm and happiness. They will have taught themselves to practice mindfulness or have frequent quiet time. Living in the now is a way of life in which acceptance plays a major role. It also requires compassion and a lack of judgment: not always having opinions, thoughts, or feelings about everything. What remains is, simply, *consciously being* in the moment. Such an attitude to life is a buffer against stress and tension. Living in the now is not about having a sense of time, but about surrendering to time. It's a state of consciousness rather than life without a clock, in which you learn to recognize that you *are not* your thoughts, but you *have* thoughts. The trick is not to have *more* control over those thoughts but rather to ease up on them and not give them too much weight—here and now is where you are.

A remarkable added benefit of having a loved one with dementia is that they can be a teacher when it comes to living in the now. While their expertise may not be the outcome of intensive practice but the result of an illness, people with dementia show us what it means to be present. They gradually transform from human doings into human beings. My mother is no longer consciously concerned with what was said last week or what's on the agenda next month. When I'm with her, the present moment is all there is. When I go and see her with a head full of noise—*Don't forget to wash the boys' soccer jerseys; Oh, and make sure you fill up the car*; and *Did I say something weird to my colleague at that meeting?*—I'm incapable of concentrating on her. None of those worries and anxieties matter when I'm with her; in fact, they only get in the way of real contact. There's a saying from Zen Buddhism: When you're hungry, eat; when you're thirsty, drink; when you're tired, sleep. It means do what has to be done here and now. That's what life is all about. Direct your attention to what needs your attention right now.

I don't want to romanticize it. It's not as if every time I visit, my mother is sitting by the window like a calm, happy Buddha, bathed in sunlight. But no matter how she feels, I can't be anywhere with my thoughts except with her. She inspires stillness in me. When it's nice and peaceful in the now, I enjoy reading to her or we'll listen to music together. But sometimes it's sad in the now, and I'm unable to get through to her or she sees things that are invisible to me. What I'm learning is that everything is always in flux, flowing, meandering. Things come and go. I often think of the quote by Theodore Roosevelt, "Do what you can, with what you have, where you are." For her that way of life is the end point, for me the starting point, and we meet halfway down that path. The ephemeral and the eternal dance together, and we try to keep up with the steps.

In his book on dementia, Huub Buijssen writes about the sense of past and present.

> *In the course of this phase, the person with dementia will experience the so-called basic feelings only: disgust, sadness, anxiety, pleasure, and trust. Any feelings that call for careful, premeditated thought disappear. Shame or regret imply knowledge of prevailing standards, and in order to show admiration and gratitude, we need to comprehend what someone's achievement has entailed.*
>
> *The person with dementia also has no more feelings relating to either the past or the future. How can he foster hope, if the future no longer exists for him. How can he feel revenge if he cannot remember what another did to him? And how can he feel guilt or remorse about something he has long forgotten?*
>
> *It is in this phase, therefore, that the person with dementia loses all contact with feelings such as shame, gratitude, guilt, hope, revenge, and remorse.*

I don't see the loss of one's sense of past and future and the ability to live in the now as some form of enlightenment. Like other emotions, shame and remorse are part of our inner compass, necessary tools for navigating life. They help us to hold our own in social interactions or provide a stimulus for growth and development. When such feelings or one's sense of time disappear, all kinds of important road markers fall by the wayside as well.

What I'm trying to say is this: Dementia really puts the way we're guided (and sidetracked) by thoughts and feelings, by time and urgency, into perspective. My mother teaches me to observe more closely. Let's face it, how often are our reactions colored by our *thoughts* about something rather than what's actually in front of us? It's a strange paradox, and this is the lesson I'm drawing from my mom's illness. The dementia of a loved one can make us more *alert*, as well as more grateful for the things we once took for granted, more mindful of what really matters, more relaxed about everyday pressures, and more present in the moment. My mother reminds me of the magic of a tender touch, the pleasure in tasting a fresh strawberry, sitting down together, a genuine smile.

The downside of the present is that you can become trapped in it. As a (primary) caregiver, especially, there'll be times when you drown in the moment, because there seems to be precious little time or space to look back or to look beyond today. Your day-to-day cares can rob you of all perspective, leaving life in the now feeling mostly stressful and exhausting. This hopelessness and sense of being stuck also affected my father and the rest of the family. One occasion, when my mother still lived at home, stands out. It was late, and she was already asleep. I'd stayed with her that evening, so my father could attend choir practice, safe in the knowledge that she'd be all right. On his return, we drank a glass of wine together, and the conversation turned to hopes and dreams for the future. At that point, he couldn't imagine that one day life might involve anything other than helping my mother 24-7. Every morning, he'd open the curtains on the present day; he never looked beyond that. He had let go of his dreams of foreign travel, museum visits, and outings with his grandchildren. It upset me that my father had become so trapped. Soon after, I gave him a little piggy bank for his birthday. It was a symbolic gift, an invitation to invest in the future. "Not now doesn't mean not ever," I told him.

Less than a year later, my father, brothers, and I were standing in Times Square in New York, the city he'd been so eager to see for himself and a trip he hadn't thought was possible. By then my mother was no longer living at home, and the grief over her admission was still fresh. But with other people now sharing our caregiving responsibilities, the four of us were able to get away. We don't know what lies ahead but entertaining the possibility that there may be something good or beautiful in the future, in spite of everything, is called hope.

And here's how we come full circle: There's always hope in the now. Hoping begins with exploring what you're feeling and experiencing right now before imagining how life may be easier or better. By doing little things, you gradually move, step by step, in that direction. And you keep moving. The more often you choose a hopeful thought, the more you dare to imagine the good things that may be in the pipeline, and the more you train your mind to focus on opportunities and possibilities—and, when they arise, to act accordingly.

In due course, hope becomes a natural, instinctive way of life and you learn to trust that however tiny your steps may be, they can have a positive impact. What's so remarkable about hope is that it's something you can learn. Hope may *feel* like an emotion, but it's actually a mindset—one in which you open up to the idea that there are possibilities that you can't envision right now. But if you keep moving, gently yet powerfully, you will always get past the moment you're stuck in right now.

LETTING GO OF THE EGO

We're walking down the corridors of my mother's home. She's taking such big strides that I can't keep up with her. "Mom, wait!" I say, laughing. No reaction. "Mom, please, slow down!" I shout a bit louder. Still no response. Then I call her by her first name. She stops and turns around. On the face of it, this may seem like an insignificant moment, but a tiny crack appears in my heart. I realize that she no longer feels spoken to when I call her "Mom." She doesn't realize that by calling her Mom, as I have done for over forty years, I'm appealing to the unique bond between us: She's my mother; I'm her only daughter. If she no longer recognizes my "Mom" as coming from her own daughter, then who am I? What's your role onstage when your costar has forgotten hers?

"Egolessness." I have chosen this word as the umbrella term for letting go of expectations and longings that originate within myself. The literal translation of the Latin *ego* is "I" or "self," and it is this self that must be abandoned, the way you perceive yourself, which is shaped in large part by your roles in life, including those of child, partner, or sibling.

The word "ego" is often shrouded in negative connotations, and it's true that somebody with a big ego and without the capacity for self-reflection can grate on your nerves. The inflated ego of a self-satisfied and selfish person leaves little room for others; however, I'm using it as a more neutral term for the self, for identity, for the thoughts we have about our individuality and our place in the world.

Even though my mother is the one with dementia, her illness means that I'm surrendering parts of my identity, too. While her "self" is changing, the "selves" of those around her are also transforming in the process: my brothers and I as her children, my father as her partner. This raises new questions about our identity. For instance, are you still somebody's child when that person no longer identifies as your mother? The first time my mother clearly didn't recognize me, I noticed that besides pain I also felt some shame. I hadn't yet met the caregiver who was on the ward at the time, so she didn't know me as a family member. To all the people in that room, I was "nobody." Never before had I been a stranger in the same space as a blood relative, and when you come from a close-knit family, like I do, that's a particularly strange sensation. In fact, it almost brought out the belligerent kid in me. Wait a minute, I know her better than anyone else around here! My ego was whimpering, and my higher self had to appease the situation.

When it comes to dementia, this egolessness can be pushed to the limits at times. I remember reading a book of interviews with well-known Dutch people about the dementia of their nearest and dearest. One of them is quoted as saying about the relationship with his father: "When the mind dissolves and the memories fade, that intimate bond you have with someone disappears, too." It was said about his father's death, though the same can be said about dementia. Although I can relate to this and I understand how sad it is when a special relationship is fundamentally changed by dementia, to me it yet again stresses the meaning and importance of egolessness. Does my mother's life cease to be precious when I can no longer experience the intimacy we once had? Surely it's not up to someone else, whoever it may be, to confirm who we are?

I could have opted for the word "selfless." When you are selfless, it is easier to focus on another person's needs. This is the perennial challenge when I'm with my mother. I must admit that in the beginning, especially, I tended to give her instructions. "Sit down now," I'd say, when she got to her feet again. Or, "We were heading this way," when, halfway through a walk, she'd turn on her heels and walk in the other direction. At some point, I realized that I was too domineering. Why would she have to sit down, or why did I insist we go on walking in the original direction? What if I were to follow *her*? What if I put myself fully at her disposal and let go of my own expectations? It would give me peace and freedom, and I think it would do the same for her.

I leave my ego at the door. We don't have to go down the same old route, nor do we have to tread familiar ground. Those who love somebody with dementia will have to learn to put themselves at the other person's service. Maybe I can do something for her: console her, alleviate any discomfort, ease her pain. My mother brings out all the tenderness in me. You'd be hard-pressed to show your love in a purer, more genuine way.

Adelheid Roosen, a Dutch actor, playwright, and documentary filmmaker, is a great example of someone who can let go of her ego when it comes to dealing with dementia. "I exist because you exist" is her starting point. She has mastered the art of completely tuning in to the needs of the other person—in her case her mother who's living with Alzheimer's. Her documentary *Mam* ("Mom") contains many moving scenes, including one in which she's taking a bath with her mother.

It's truly remarkable. Roosen was able to completely immerse herself in her mother's world, probably because, as a trained actor, she's used to playing other characters. Perhaps we can't all go as far as she was able to, but I suspect that there's a little bit of that skill in each of us. Roosen is known as the "Alzheimer's whisperer," as she has translated her personal insights into practical tips for all those dealing with the disease, either professionally or privately.

One of those pointers is dare to be shameless. Shake off your embarrassment and go crazy. It's not as hard as we sometimes think, even if there may be a mental barrier stopping you from, say, dancing among adults with dementia. My elder brother once walked into my mother's nursing home during a disco event. Before her illness, my mom wasn't a regular on the dance floor, and my brother—let's just say that he isn't the type to embrace that kind of thing, yet he didn't hesitate to unleash his inner John Travolta.

I read an interview with Adelheid Roosen in which she says something lovely about her mother's inability to recognize her: "She remembers me, but she doesn't always know what a daughter is. . . . Yet she remembers me as something that's part of her being. Something familiar." That's so beautiful! I find it touching, because the same is true for my mom. She recognizes us on a much deeper level. We can tell from the way she leans into hugs or initiates contact. Being unknown is not the same as being a stranger, and that's comforting.

"I know what you're trying to say," I tell my brother. I hear his hesitation on the other end of the line, in the absence of language. It's a silence that's not uncommon between us, and I know exactly which piece of the puzzle fits in it, which words we're not saying out loud. And sometimes we do articulate them, and then we fall silent afterward, because we're thinking the same thing: When will we have to let her go for good?

On several occasions now my mom has come dangerously close to the edge, because something in her body was malfunctioning or failing altogether. Each time it puts us in a state of high alert. We want to rush over to my mother and make sure that my father receives the necessary support. Up until now, it has always been a false alarm, and she has managed to claw her way back to life. Sometimes it feels like we're doing test runs for when the actual moment arrives.

As the caregiver of a person with dementia, you may be familiar with this scenario. It's always there in the background, as a latent possibility—the moment when our loved one slips away. The incurable, progressive disease will catch up with her one day. Until then, we won't know exactly when or how it will happen. My mother is like a sandcastle in the surf. One by one, the waves of time wash over it. At times something fundamental disappears into the depths, at others the swell is barely visible, but she'll be washed away. That's unavoidable.

It's hard to say this out loud, let alone write down, but sometimes we tell each other it's all right if she goes. While she still enjoys a good quality of life—has moments without pain and suffering but with peace of mind, fun, and happiness—we'll look after her to the very best of our ability. But whenever she's feeling ill or unsettled, we'd love to be able to spare her that brutally long decline that she herself would have abhorred. The paradox of death in dementia is that it would break our hearts, but also give us comfort. It's a full stop, an end to her ordeal. I almost want that for her. I wish she were able to let go of her earthly body, which is so bravely trying to keep her here but is increasingly ill-equipped to provide her with a safe home.

It's painful to admit, because what kind of person would say that she could come to terms with her mother dying? What does that say about you? But death can be a deliverance. There comes a time when enough is enough. When I think of that moment, tears stream down my face. But then again, the tears are also rolling down my cheeks while I sit with her when she's unwell or struggling. She's like a little bird under the thick covers, so fragile, so vulnerable, her eyes so distant. If she'd have wanted to slip away in one of those moments, I'd have summoned all the love I have in me and not tried to keep her here.

I'm moved by the words of Nicci Gerrard about death and dementia.

And yet death can also restore a person, especially when that person had been unmade by dementia. Once they die, they are no longer only old and frail and ill, they are no longer only confused and forgetful, no longer a wrecked body and a failing mind, no longer not themselves. Because they have gone from us, they can come back to us and be all the selves they have ever been. Young, old, everything in between. Robust, vulnerable, everything in between. And often we fall head over heels in love with all these selves and we understand how they contained multitudes.

It's a beautiful thought, this release, this healing. Death isn't just something to fear, it's also a relief. I've noticed that my father, who loves my mother with every fiber of his being, has been thinking about this, too. Part of him dreads it, and that fear rises every time there's a crisis. But as long as he sees that she still gets some joy out of life, as does he, he clings to the idea that they can probably maintain this way of being for a while longer. Yet when I press him on it, he acknowledges that there's no such thing as a status quo in dementia. So we keep a close eye on her, her rhythm, her body and soul, and in the meantime we do what we can: ensure that she's not in pain, that she's comfortable and warm, and that she feels safe and secure.

Some believe in an afterlife, a place where everything that hurts will drop away from us. The body is a temporary shell for the soul, which after death will evolve into something intangible. Others believe in reincarnation, the transition to a new life form. I think my mother believed in some form of heaven. Perhaps she's already on her way to a place where she's free and light. The tender comfort that emanates from that idea warms my heart—I really want to believe it with her.

What's so comforting about "deliverance" is that it means "the state of being saved from a painful or bad experience." It has the same root as "delivery," the moment when a baby enters this world, pure and unblemished, to take its place among us. In religious parlance, the word "deliverance" is used to indicate that somebody has put their sins behind them and is once again righteous and pure. Deliverance marks the end of grief and suffering and the beginning of purity and a clean slate. Death as just such a release soothes my heart.

THE SILVER LININGS
ALONG THE WAY

LOVE AND OTHER TENDER COMFORTS

Unconditional love is selfless love—without deriving any benefit from it yourself. Giving somebody your love without expecting anything in return demands a very big and open heart. Although more challenging than it looks on paper, pure, unconditional love is a huge gift that you can give at any moment. Compared to those who don't experience this kind of love, people who are loved in this way feel more secure, autonomous, and confident, which is all highly beneficial for the immune system. Knowing yourself to be loved, even though you're making mistakes, changing, or are no longer capable of being an equal partner in the relationship significantly enhances your quality of life. Love is particularly welcome when we suffer. Among other things, it releases oxytocin, which you may know as the "love hormone" and which boosts your mood and sense of connection—especially when coupled with a hug or a kiss. And let's face it, all people with dementia need love.

When a loved one is diagnosed with dementia, your relationship will undoubtedly change. In the case of romantic love the partner relationship may be lost, the roles in a parent–child relationship will be reversed, and in close friendships much of your common ground will disappear altogether. Being on the front line of caregiving forces you to explore just what "unconditional" really means, as you can't always count on gratitude, cooperation, recognition, or compensation. It's important to remember that unconditional isn't the same as unlimited or unequal. In an ongoing (care) relationship, you can't give indefinitely; sooner or later you're going to run out of steam. For that reason, you should also love *yourself* unconditionally—no more or less, but just as much.

Can you love somebody when that person no longer responds to your love? I think it's possible to love unconditionally when the object of your love has dementia. A special characteristic of love is that it puts a glow in your own heart before you can give it away. You can't bestow it without feeling it yourself first. The wise Buddhist nun Pema Chödrön puts it like this: "When you begin to *touch* your *heart* or let your *heart* be *touched*, you begin to discover that it's bottomless, that it doesn't have any resolution, that this heart is huge, vast, and limitless." Our heart is immense, bigger than you could possibly imagine.

The vagus nerve is one of our longest nerves and is responsible for carrying information to and from the brain and organs. Also known as "the link between body and mind," it is thought to sync in people who love each other deeply, helping them pick up on each other's emotions and even synchronizing the rhythm of their heartbeats. This process make you responsive and sensitive to the other's well-being, and it's also good for your own health. Two hearts beating as one, isn't that both a magical and a comforting idea? When your loved one with dementia can sense your love at that level you can make a real difference and include them in that love by expressing your warmth and affection, even by merely *feeling* it.

My father and I wrote a line from *The Little Prince* by Antoine de Saint-Exupéry on last year's Christmas cards to my mother's caregivers: "It is only with the heart that one can see rightly; what is essential is invisible to the eye." As described previously, in its early stages, dementia is mostly confined to the outer layer of the brain, while the deeper, emotional centers remain unimpaired for a long time. When the thinking mind is damaged, feelings grow stronger and more intense—and that includes the experience of love. It may be all but imperceptible in the way they behave or what they say, but rest assured: Your love still matters, your love is felt.

When a loved one has dementia you may suddenly find yourself receiving the love that wasn't readily expressed before. A friend told me about her father who used to be quick to voice his disapproval, whether it be the major she chose in college, the friends she hung out with, or the city she moved to. But over time, dementia softened his intransigence and revealed his pride and warmth—now his pure, unbridled paternal love makes her feel more like his daughter than ever. Sadly, dementia can also result in the opposite, with your loved one forgetting that you occupy a special place in her heart. This can be particularly painful for partners, for example when their other half becomes infatuated with a fellow patient.

I must admit that in the name of love for my mother, and occasionally both parents, my brothers and I have made decisions that didn't feel like an act of love to them at all. I contacted their family doctor without their consent, arranged for caregivers to come in, and later decided that my mom could no longer stay at home. It falls under the banner of what we call "tough love." Tough love is having the courage to navigate toward unsentimental decisions, which are ultimately in the other person's most loving interest. Love makes us courageous and brave; it's the fuel we need to overcome practical or emotional barriers, because we only want the best for each other. Love can be a driving force for change because it gives us the strength to navigate high mountains as well as deep troughs.

Hindu culture believes that we all have an energy body with various focal points known as "chakras." Your heart has such an energy point, too. In Sanskrit it's called *Anahata*, which means "unhurt." Your heart is the place where you're whole and complete, where you can't be touched by dementia itself or by worries about your loved one's illness. It's the line between you that will always be open.

If you see the heart as a place from which to connect, why don't you rest your hand on your heart as a reminder when you're talking or thinking about someone. Straighten your back and drop your shoulders, so your chest feels relaxed and open. Gently breathe in and out to slow your pulse and keep opening your heart to those you love, time and time again.

My mother isn't always good at expressing her love, especially not now that she has been robbed of her language. But there are moments when the affection is back, as if all the stars are magically aligned. She'll sit up with a look of recognition and the most radiant smile you can imagine. Hey, Mom! There you are. Even when I fail to get a reaction, we still speak the universal language of the heart that keeps us connected. I remind myself that she loves me, whether she can say so or not. It brings to mind a passage from the book *Still Alice* by Lisa Genova, in which the protagonist with Alzheimer's says, "Love is safe from the mayhem of the mind, because it lives in our hearts."

I often talk to my children about the "silver thread." About how they were attached to me by a thick silver cord, a magic cord, when they were born, which subsequently transformed into an invisible and unbreakable silver thread that will tie us together forever. Whenever they feel alone, all they have to do is think of that delicate thread and we're connected. I picture a similar silver thread between me and my mother.

I trust that her memories of the two of us together and her love for me are like Atlantis, lying on the ocean bed, just below the surface. I'm sustained by the subtlety of love: a smile, a hug, seeing her relax in my company, and knowing that she sometimes reaches for me and allows my kisses.

Love is something we don't forget.

I cherish her as the mother she was *and* the one she is now, and it is unconditional love that helped me get to this stage. I want to love her and fully embrace her, together with the dementia that has befallen her. With his huge heart, my father lives and breathes unconditional love in everything he does. In spite of it all, he still sees the young woman he promised to love and cherish for better or worse. Witnessing that kind of love ultimately has an impact on all the relationships you have and value in your life; it filters through in the contact with all those you connect with. Learning to love unconditionally, through trial and error, is one of dementia's unexpected gifts.

In an interview with a Dutch magazine, Marianne Williamson said something about love that has always stayed with me: "We all labor under the illusion that life is long and love short. In fact, it's the other way around: Love is eternal and life brief. People come and go. But love lasts if you keep on loving. Love is an adventure of the soul. Dedicate as much time and energy as possible to love."

Small acts of love

- Keep addressing your loved one as an adult human being in their own right.
- Communicate your love by saying "I like you" or "I love you."
- Express yourself through body language with a smile, open arms, or by leaning forward.
- Draw on all your senses, including taste and touch. Be gentle.
- Frequently touch the other person.
- Talk about favorite subjects.
- Offer friendly encouragement such as "Well done!"
- Provide comfort by simply being there.
- Be patient and allow for plenty of time.
- Take the other person's emotions and behavior seriously.
- Share memories about highlights.

HUMOR

I'm in the lobby of my mother's nursing home, waiting for my meeting with the social worker. The reception area doubles as a restaurant and is always a lively place. It's the backdrop to many entertaining episodes between the colorful characters that pass through: residents, visitors, and caregivers alike.

Four people are playing cards at a nearby table. Sitting next to them are a resident and his visitor. I overhear their conversation. One of the card players asks the guy at the other table: "Who are you?"

The other resident: "Who, me?"

His visitor: "This is Nick."

Nick himself: "Who's Nick?"

"You are!"

"Who?"

"Nick!"

"Says who?'"

"I do."

"Oh, all right then, if you say so."

It makes me laugh, this droll exchange in response to what is, to a healthy brain, a straightforward question. It's funny when people express themselves a little clumsily. Humor is a universal, timeless language. It can connect people and cut right across the dementia. For a long time, I was able to bond with my mother and get her attention by imitating my father's way of speaking. The two of us would laugh about him behind his back. She enjoyed that. A joke can inject a bit of much-needed air and light. My mom's caregivers frequently deploy humor, too, because it can defuse an unpleasant situation, brighten her mood, and make a medical procedure easier. When she has to be hoisted into bed, it's more fun if the caregiver does it with a big wink: "Right, here you go again!" And if you want her to maintain muscle strength, why not encourage her to move by suggesting a little dance to a cheerful tune.

I don't know anything better than humor at blowing some air into situations that feel heavy and dark. Quite literally a laugh requires a deep breath. Laughter is good for your physical well-being—it relaxes your muscles, lowers your blood pressure, and produces endorphins and serotonin, the body's natural painkillers. Laughter is also good for your mental health. It helps you put things into perspective, pulls you into the present, and enables you to see a new angle. The side effects of a genuine smile are beneficial to both you and your loved one. With the diagnosis and the actual illness beset with worry and sadness, it's all but essential to offset by celebrating the brighter side of life. There are enough dark moments.

It may feel paradoxical to have fun when there's not a lot to laugh about. Still, you should allow for that levity. It really helps to alleviate stress and tension, and it is a useful coping mechanism that can make the difference between a bad day and a good one. In an interview on the podcast *Fresh Air*, Stephen Colbert spoke of humor as an antidote to potentially paralyzing fear and difficult emotions. He said, "You can't *laugh* and be *afraid* at the same time." It's a beautiful way of saying that humor provides distraction and allows you to briefly rise above the situation.

Humor also strengthens the bond between those who are in on the joke. It's an effective way of creating and maintaining mutual trust. Even when other forms of communication are changing or falling away with dementia, humor will continue to provide an effective method of connection. As long as it's genuine—and you're laughing *with*, not *at*, someone—there's no reason not to occasionally burst out laughing.

My brothers and I often resort to humor to ease our own sadness or discomfort. We never feel guilty about it, because we know that it's done with the greatest respect for our mother and her dementia. We desperately need our jokes for emotional release. We can laugh in the safety of our mutual trust and shared sense of wit. When it comes to humor, tastes certainly differ (and change over time). Everybody—with or without dementia—has their own laughter triggers. These days, my mother even laughs at visiting clowns who draw soapy hearts on windows, whereas I'm pretty sure that this clownish comedy wouldn't have been her thing in the past. But who cares?

When you feel that you don't have much to laugh about, I recommend actively seeking out what might tickle you. Maybe it's a clip of a particular stand-up comedian or entertainer; perhaps it's a funny movie that helps you relax; or, if you have a penchant for darker humor, it might be satire that sets you off. On one website about dementia, I came across a well-worn joke: "What's the advantage of dementia? You can hide your own Easter eggs!" That made me chuckle.

If we couldn't laugh, we would all go insane.

CONNECTEDNESS

Connection comes in unexpected places. One afternoon a new caregiver welcomed us at our mother's home with open, visibly tattooed arms. She had pink hair with an undercut on one side. I remember my brother and I looking at each other: "Right, let's see Mom's reaction." My mother had never been a big fan of that kind of look; when my brother and I dyed our hair bluish black she wasn't impressed, to put it mildly. And, according to her, having my ears pierced a second time was an example of "extreme piercing." But this particular caregiver ended up becoming not just her favorite, but the whole family's. The dementia has had the positive side effect of making my parents realize, more than ever, that those things are not all that relevant. It's not about "looking respectable" or coloring inside the lines. What matters is that there are people who open their arms to you, reach out, and make you feel safe and at home, even when you're not there by choice.

We need one another. The web we form together is all around us. Our lives are closely intertwined; nobody can go it alone. Even on a purely biological level, we need others to maintain our best possible mental and physical health. Our nervous system is more responsive to stress in isolation than in connection with others. People are naturally social beings, herd animals. We seek one another's company, in clubs and teams and neighborhoods and cities, however much we long to spend time on our own every now and then.

The weird thing is that we often forget just *how* connected we are. We take for granted what is actually human-made or has passed through human hands, from the bread we eat and the medication we take to the blankets we sleep under. Nothing in life is not connected to something or somebody else. Even the self exists because of others and those others because of us. But now that our lives are becoming increasingly disconnected and mediated via screens, we often look without seeing and hear without listening. That's not good enough when the chips are down. Dementia forces us to take a step back and *really* connect and be present.

We all want to have a place in the world. Our self-awareness and self-worth are tied up in feeling useful. The best way to keep nurturing our connection with life is by continuing to be a functional part of it. The caregivers on my mother's ward have recently started cooking fresh meals from scratch. Something as ordinary and simple as chopping up a tomato or cooking pasta (or feeling that you're lending a helping hand) can give you a sense of belonging.

Paradoxical as it may sound, a connection with others is necessary if you want to retain your autonomy. Like the rest of us, a person with dementia wants to experience a degree of independence, and yet the illness makes this impossible. That's why they need others to help bolster a sense of autonomy as the dementia progresses. For us to feel independent, we need others to acknowledge our independence. We experience freedom through connectedness.

Unfortunately, dementia is often a source of loneliness and isolation. Somewhere down the road, close friends and relatives will disappear. When a relationship is no longer experienced as equal or the initiative to reach out becomes more and more one-sided, valuable connections die a slow death. Add to this the ignorance about the disease and fear of the unknown, and there are many great losses. Most people don't withdraw on purpose or with any malicious intent, but out of sheer powerlessness. And you may find that this doesn't just happen to the patient but also to you in your own social life.

As a caregiver, you may feel a suffocating loneliness behind closed doors, because people have no idea how demanding your days are. Loneliness isn't uncommon in the second line of care, either. You're experiencing something that others don't understand or recognize, and it feels like you're living under a bell jar. You can look out but sense an invisible barrier between your life and that of others. A combination of powerlessness, apparent hopelessness, and loneliness can bring even the strongest to their knees.

The more stories I've heard from people who have a loved one with dementia, the more I've come to realize that we're *not* alone in my mother's illness. Knowing this gives me strength and comfort and further underlines the importance of sharing and being honest about our experiences—this book is my way of reaching out.

We may have this great fear of dependency . . . but depending on one another isn't the end of the world. I've certainly come to understand that it's also a blessing of sorts. I'm grateful that the dementia has made the bond between me and my family more palpable than ever. My relationship with my father and brothers has only deepened. It's not that we always agree or think along the same lines, but by holding one another tight we stay strong and are able to endure more than we could on our own. One of my brothers takes care of financial and administrative tasks, the other tidies up our father's house from time to time and cleans the kitchen. I buy clothes for my mother. We listen to one another and laugh and cry together. I wear my mother's ring with the five small diamonds in a row (one for each of our families), because as the driving force behind our unity she remains an integral part of our family.

Have you lost that sense of connectedness? Then it's a good idea to go out and do something that makes you feel part of a greater whole again. You could visit a museum or attend a concert, join a club, invite a neighbor for coffee, or join a Facebook group. When you feel cut off from the rest of the world, you're not in the best position to handle adversity.

It's also incredibly important to know people who are in the same boat. We can learn from one another, and as we're going through more or less the same thing we speak the same language. People with a loved one with advanced dementia can draw on their inside knowledge to share what steps they had to take, while newcomers to the illness can speak to those who know what they're talking about. It's very satisfying to be of use to others. My father dreaded the prospect of a support group, but we convinced him to attend one—and he found comfort and recognition. It may feel like we're alone, but in reality we never are.

WHAT REALLY MATTERS

When dementia crosses our path, everything is thrown into sharp focus. We start noticing what's not going well, what's changing, what's going wrong, and what may bring (more) pain and grief. It's what any form of danger does to our brain. This instinctive, almost unconscious, alertness is an evolutionary response to potential threats to our survival. It can, however, render us blind to all the other things that matter—everything that continues to go well, the relaxing moments, the twinkles of love. Small as they may be, the good, the light, and the pleasant are also worth noticing. They're the bright spots in what often feels like a dark tunnel. As the saying widely attributed to a Chinese proverb goes, "It is better to light a single candle than to curse the darkness." Dementia can be a lens through which to view the world around you differently, in more detail, with more nuance. It's a lens that gives you a crystal-clear vision of pain and sadness, as well as love and happiness. Dementia shows you what's essential.

Anyone who aspires to a pure and simple life will find inspiration in a person with dementia. My mother no longer cares about what I'm wearing, whether or not I'm successful, or what mistakes I've made. Ultimately your appearance, mistakes, relationships, and most other things don't matter in dementia. In the end, not even the gifts you bring, the length of your visits, or your ability to afford extra care have any value. What really counts is what lies beneath: the sincerity of your intentions, your undivided attention, your palpable love, and showing up without being intent on a particular outcome or result.

Psychologists have found that people can be categorized into *maximizers* and *satisficers* (combining the words "satisfy" and "suffice"). For the first group, only the very best will do, while the second is content with good enough. It turns out that people who are prepared to compromise are happier. Not obsessing about success or appearance helps you avoid feelings of unrest and stress. The better you are at modifying your expectations, dealing with disappointment, and letting go of the desire to control everything, the closer you come to what really matters. You can then fill the space that's freed up and the time you save with attention, love, and meaning.

My mother reminds me over and over that some things are simply not as important as I sometimes think. Have I washed my hair? What vase should the flowers go in? What are my vacation plans? Having said that, some issues will always matter. If the circumstances are *not* conducive to rest and relaxation for either you or your loved one, then you have to do something about it. When your loved one's environment is safe and pleasant, it may clear the way for more visits, for example. What matters is the comfort of your loved one. Are they safe? Are they relaxed? The rest is noise. Let's not lose sight of what's important in dementia: tenderness, an open heart, and trust. And the courage to keep returning, again and again, to what really matters. The trick is to feel pain but not turn away from it; to feel sadness, but not allow yourself to be eaten up by it; to feel love and appreciate the moment.

GRATITUDE

When caring for somebody with dementia, you give a lot: your time, your attention, your resources, your energy. It may feel natural that people turn to you for help—you can't imagine *not* being available; of course, you'll do what you can, you have no choice. In a caregiving relationship, the focus is often entirely on giving, which makes sense. But even when there's no dementia, many people find it easier to give than to receive.

Balancing between giving and receiving to avoid burn-out seems straightforward enough on paper. But what does receiving mean in the context of dementia? This calls for some mental gymnastics. Receive what? From whom? When you're in the first circle around the patient, you'll probably feel that there isn't much of a balance. At times the endless giving will feel like a huge, inescapable burden.

To rebalance the situation and lighten your load, it may help to practice gratitude. It's a loaded concept in our culture because many of us were raised with enforced gratitude. You may have been told to kneel down and give thanks for the bread on the table or a roof over your head. It was a way of stifling ambition and desire. I can't think of anything positive about thankfulness as a passive, submissive approach to life. My mother's dementia—I should be grateful for *that*? The fact that my mother won't see my children grow up, that we can't have a conversation even though she's sitting right next to me, that we can only watch as her body and thinking mind are slowly erased? No, thanks. I'll pass.

And yet my mother's illness has deepened my approach to gratitude. In its purest form, gratefulness can furnish dark clouds with silver linings. Stripped of all negative cultural connotations, practicing gratitude is a proven method for helping you feel calmer and happier amid everything that's going on. Many studies have shown that people who practice gratitude feel better and more positive. It boosts the immune system, increases your self-confidence, and helps you sleep better. Gratitude reminds you to stay focused on the good, especially while navigating the deepest lows and the darkest days. When we struggle to deal with the big issues in life, it's all the more important to be thankful for the little things.

I try to identify at least three things I'm grateful for every day. It shines a light on the nice things in my life while my mother is ill. Dementia comes with good and beautiful moments that we'll only notice if we pay attention. There may even be occasions for pride. A friend told me that she's incredibly proud of her father, who recently moved into an assisted-living facility. Having previously sworn never to leave his own home, he now accepts his new place with calm and composure. Her father is more flexible than she ever could have imagined. I recognize this, too: I'm proud of my mother when she cracks jokes with the caregivers and when she's strong enough to overcome yet another setback. That's when I think to myself, look at her, she's doing amazing.

Itemizing everything I'm grateful for feels like an expression of love for my mother and enables me to look beyond the dementia. I'm thankful when she can enjoy music or good food. I'm thankful that my parents love each other so much. I'm thankful that my mom is so well looked after. I'm thankful that I can handle so much more than I thought I could. I'm thankful that my heart is capable of unconditional love.

And who are we supposed to be grateful to? You can express gratitude even if God has no place in your life. We receive from life itself. We're dependent on everything and everybody on this planet, from the trees releasing oxygen to the water that makes life possible, from our parents who bring us into this world to the sun that rises in the morning. We receive so we can live. Even gratitude that's not addressed to anything or anyone will always find its place.

MASKS OFF

We're always making subtle adjustments to situations, people, and circumstances. At work you're likely more thoughtful about what you say than you are at the kitchen table with friends. You're more likely to verbally lash out at a loved one than at a stranger. You dress better for a wedding than for the weekly grocery run. We learn to adjust to the circumstance as children, otherwise we risk being ostracized. From a purely evolutionary standpoint, fitting in is important for survival. But when we enter the world of dementia, these masks often fall by the wayside. Ingrained patterns and learned behavior may change, disappear, or become exaggerated, which can transform the dynamic between you and your loved one.

When someone no longer has to obey certain rules, we may well see that person begin to thrive. I've heard stories of people suddenly becoming quite carefree and laid-back after a lifetime of hard work, and those who used to be distant and hard becoming mellow and growing more affectionate. If anything, I've seen my mother become more relaxed as the dementia has advanced. Once she no longer had to (or could) put up a brave front, she found it easier to take each day as it came.

The moment everything that we rely on to shape and prop up our identity falls away, we can see one another for the mortal human beings that we are. The noise fades to make way for authenticity. Groups of people who find themselves in high-pressured situations will often develop a great sense of connection and unity. When the chips are down, there's not a lot of space for ego tripping or games. In vulnerability you have to show yourself for who you really are, and that leads to *true* intimacy, solidarity, and trust.

But there's no guarantee of positive transformation. Dementia can also bring about insidious, painful changes that have an alienating effect. Some people become mean, suspicious, or aggressive. In which case, was *this* your loved one's pure essence all along, hidden behind a mask? No. Let's not forget that dementia can cause shifts in personality and inexplicable behaviors that will make you feel that people are further from their real self rather than closer to it. Besides, a person with dementia will experience daily mood swings, just like everybody else. Dementia is a complex disease with symptoms that vary depending on the area of the brain that's affected and the experiences somebody has had throughout their life. Combined with a lack of inhibition triggered by dementia, this can manifest in an unpleasant way. It's incredibly difficult and sad when this happens to your loved one. I'm sorry that you're going through this. Your experience needs to be acknowledged and seen, too.

Maybe the only comfort lies in the knowledge that, as the illness progresses, this stage will pass again. An acquaintance told me that her mother's worsening dementia was a blessing in disguise because it took away her difficult behavior. That, too, is the reality of dementia.

In a beautiful metaphor, the spiritual teacher Ram Dass compares people to trees. He writes that when you look at trees and see how different they are, you accept it and appreciate those trees as they are. We don't extend this openness to humans and have a tendency to judge them. "And so I practice turning people into trees. Which means appreciating them just the way they are."

To live our lives authentically, we often need to lose something first, a veil or a mask. Drop that mask and what remains is authenticity. My mother is teaching me how I, too, can live without masks. I don't have to assume any roles when I'm with her; now that she's in a care facility, I don't even have to be a caregiver anymore. When she needs to have her clothes changed or has to use the bathroom, the caregivers at her nursing home will take over, lovingly even. Not because I can't or don't want to help her myself but because their approach is this: You just sit back, it's enough for you to simply *be* here. That's special to me, and it leaves a lot of room for genuine contact and quality time with my mother.

Behind our masks, we're all vulnerable. People who are in the same position as I am have told me moving stories about dementia fostering purity, and the suffering of others bringing us closer to our innermost selves. One of them said:

> When I'm standing by my mother's bedside, all my love and kindness come to the fore. Seeing her lying there like a blank page, she has the same effect on me as a newborn baby. For a long time, I clashed with my mother, like so many women do. I used to be angry with her. But now . . . now all I feel is love. Her dementia has brought me to that part of myself, the part of me that wants to give, that wants to love and embrace her. She's no longer verbal and I'm not sure if she recognizes me, but we're fine, the two of us together. I can honestly say to her: "Mom, I love you so much, I really like being with you." Every now and then she'll flash me a gorgeous smile and I'll go home filled with tenderness. It's a real gift to me.

And a friend told me: "My brother-in-law has dementia. I'm touched and moved by him. He takes me right back to the essence of life."

SELF-CONFIDENCE

When dementia crosses your path, you need to bring so many skills and talents to the table that you're bound to discover something within yourself that you didn't know existed. Perhaps you're far better at coping with stress than you thought, or calmer, stronger, or more pragmatic. Getting to know yourself on an even deeper level is a remarkable by-product of this whole process. And that breeds self-confidence—the ability to trust your own judgment and capabilities, feeling that you can handle life, however it unfolds.

So much of what we do is done on autopilot. Anyone who's ever tried to consciously change their behavior, be it to lose weight or quit an unhealthy habit, knows how difficult and demanding it can be. That makes it truly extraordinary that we're able to change and grow. Dementia can have that effect on beholders: It helps us grow and evolve. The social worker in my mother's nursing home sees this on a daily basis. People start cooking and undertake household duties for the first time in their lives, looking after the finances, or taking the car to the mechanic. Managing all these tasks is a huge accomplishment.

In some people's eyes, you'll never get it right. There are those who'll underestimate the situation, whereas others will be keen to point out what you should be doing differently. But remember, none of them are in your shoes. Self-confidence also means trusting that you're acting in good conscience and to the best of your ability—and to stand by that, even if in hindsight you might have taken another, better approach.

Promise yourself that you will do something every day that nourishes and boosts your self-confidence. It can be as simple as giving yourself a compliment in front of the mirror or thanking yourself out loud.

"Thank you for doing the laundry."

"You're welcome, self, nice of you to mention it!"

It may sound childish but it's effective.

You can use the "www method" and ask yourself *What went well?* The idea is to come up with three answers every day. When you do this on a regular basis, you'll become more aware of positive elements and, like gratitude, this will have a favorable effect on your emotional well-being. It generates energy instead of using it up. This self-affirmation is important, because it gives you strength for the next stage of dementia, which will come no matter what. It's a way of building mental muscle. Glennon Doyle coined the phrase, "We can do hard things," which is an incredibly powerful mantra. You can do hard things. You can cope with dementia.

One way of reminding yourself to have and cherish constructive thoughts about yourself is by saying affirmations. You can do this throughout the day. Affirmations are powerful statements with a positive message. The word derives from the Latin *affirmare* and means "to strengthen" or "to corroborate." The more you repeat an affirmation, the more likely you are to make it a reality. Not because it's a magic spell, but because it helps you stay focused on what's good and beneficial for your self-confidence.

Words of affirmation

- ◆ I'm fine as I am.
- ◆ I'm doing my best and that's enough.
- ◆ I accept my feelings.
- ◆ I have an inner source of strength and love.
- ◆ I take as much time as I need.
- ◆ I'm brave.

HEALING

I can't pinpoint exactly when I reached the stage in my mother's illness when I felt that I was moving back toward the light. At some point, I realized that the dementia and I hadn't been locked in an epic struggle for some time. The disease is still there, but I'm no longer as scared or angry as I once was. That's not the same as not being sad or not feeling any pain about losing my mom, but the battle is over. Letting go of my resistance has created the space for making the remaining time worthwhile and meaningful. What's more, it has left room for healing, for picking up the pieces, and, where possible, putting them back together again, lovingly buffing the scratches and popping out the dents.

There will come a point in your loved one's dementia when you can begin to deal with what you've lost, experienced, and discovered—and I hope you're in the right headspace to get started on that now. There may be some work to do already. Whether you've only just discovered that you're going to have to accommodate dementia in your life or you've had to let your loved one go years ago—each of us has hurt inside that has yet to heal. That's all right. Healing is never completely done. What matters is not the speed but the direction in which we're traveling.

Healing means "becoming whole again," which is, crucially, not the same as "becoming your old self again." Having gone through all this, you can't simply go back to life as it was. You can only live your life going forward, starting from how you're feeling now in this moment. Doing the healing work can make you feel physically, mentally, and emotionally stronger. It will stop your energy and joie de vivre from trickling away through the cracks of life. That's why healing often reminds me of *kintsugi*, the Japanese method of repairing broken ceramics. Instead of making the breaks as invisible as possible, like nothing ever happened, the technique highlights the cracks by covering them with lacquer and gold. It gives a bowl or a cup a special and unique quality—and enables it to hold water again.

When we speak of "healing," it's not the absence of pain and grief we're aspiring to. The aim is to weave all the difficulties that the dementia has brought into the fabric of your life. But before you can do this you need to be open and honest with yourself and give your emotions a place as well as the time and attention they deserve. Kristin Neff, whose work on

WE TOO CAN REPRODUCE

OURSELVES FROM THE

SHATTERED PIECES OF

A DIFFICULT TIME.

—*Elizabeth Lesser*

compassion I quoted earlier, is right when she says: "There is *no healing without* heartwork." Emotional healing is not letting anything stop you from moving forward; it's growing, dreaming, and hoping, even if it means first acknowledging your pain and grief. Feeling pain in order to heal may seem contradictory, but another spiritual teacher, Jack Kornfield, nails it when he says, "'Free' is not free from feelings, but *free to feel* each one and let it move on, unafraid of the movement of life."

A metaphor that I like for true healing is that of the phoenix rising from the ashes. The mythical bird goes up in flames, leaving everything behind, only to emerge, reborn, from its own ashes. A phoenix is what it was, yet also wholly new; essentially the same, yet not its former self; changed, but maybe closer to its true core than ever. The spiritual teacher Elizabeth Lesser has written beautifully about the phoenix healing process.

You and I are the Phoenix. We too can reproduce ourselves from the shattered pieces of a difficult time. Our lives ask us to die and to be reborn every time we confront change—change within our self and change in our world. When we descend all the way down to the bottom of a loss, and dwell patiently, with an open heart, in the darkness and pain, we can bring back up with us the sweetness of life and the exhilaration of inner growth. When there is nothing left to lose, we find the true self— the self that is whole, the self that is enough, the self that no longer looks to others for definition, or completion, or anything but companionship on the journey.

The process of healing

The process of healing is different for us all, but there are a few common denominators. How do you know that you're healing?

- You accept that you're going through a painful process and allow yourself to really feel the emotions.
- You can stay with what you're feeling, even when it's unpleasant, because you trust that the intensity of your feelings will decrease again.
- You look after yourself in difficult times, just as you take care of others.
- You're aware that pain and happiness can take turns and complement each other.
- You feel that you're not alone, that your grief is personal to you, but not unique.
- You know which small things can make a positive difference for you.
- You are compassionate toward yourself.
- You're able to calm yourself.
- You forgive yourself for your imperfections and let the self-reproach go.
- You allow yourself to experience joy in the midst of adversity.
- You can accept help.
- You clearly identify your boundaries.

- You can name and express emotions, both to yourself and others.
- You have dreams and hopes for the future.

HAPPINESS

Even when a loved one has dementia, you have every chance and right to know happiness. You may be sad, tired, and beat; or experiencing pain, confusion, and anger, but happiness will find you.

After all my years of work and research in the field of personal growth, happiness remains as elusive as ever. But whereas I used to think that it was big and loud, I now know better. Happiness is small and intimate. It's not the constant state of being that is sold to us by advertising, films, and social media, it's not a spectacular sun-filled life without pain and grief. The simple, everyday moments of deeper connection, inner peace, and pure pleasure—they're the ones that really matter.

Life gives us little pearls of happiness to thread onto our necklace and wear close to the skin. I never thought I'd find these gems on the path of dementia, and yet I have, in connection, comfort, resilience, unconditional love. It hurts to let go of what we hold dear, but the pain is interwoven with intimacy.

Scientists tell us that some 40 percent of our happiness is determined by our genes and 10 percent by our circumstances. The remaining 50 percent is shaped by our approach to life. Isn't that comforting to know? Life may be cruel, but you still have some influence over your emotions. You don't have to be strong and positive every step of the way—you're not a robot. You've got a greater role to play in your own happiness than your feelings might suggest right now.

And you're *allowed* to be happy. Don't ever let the dementia make you forget that. When happiness comes along, in whichever form, embrace it, it's yours. Life lets flowers unfold in the most wondrous shapes, birds sing at the crack of dawn, and the evening sky light up in vivid shades of orange and pink. It's all part of the process, because beauty and perfection and joy are just as natural as storms, defects, and mortality.

You'll be honoring your loved one and the difficulties you've been through more by remaining open to happiness than by closing yourself off from it. Feeling pain isn't the same as being loyal to what you've been through, just like having fun isn't the same as disloyalty. It all exists side by side. You don't have to be perfect to be entitled to happiness.

The arrival of dementia in your life makes you feel intensely powerless. But it also presents an opportunity. When everything around you changes and you have to give up and let go of so much, you're also given a chance to take control of your life, again and again; to grow, learn, and discover. You can flesh out what really matters to you and find out just how much resilience, courage, and love you have inside of you. It's an invitation to truly embrace life, with everything you have to offer. For people who have encountered dementia, concepts like "kindness," "compassion," "surrender," and "consolation" are no longer mere words. Happy people are not the ones who never experience pain. They are those who somehow find the courage to go on living. To go on thriving.

Let the desire for happiness be your fuel. It gives us the strength to do what dementia asks of us, what life demands of us. Ultimately it boils down to opening our hearts. While this allows pain and grief to flow freely in, those same wide-open doors can also let love and comfort in. An open heart is a living heart: It has life flowing through it. When I was in New York City with my father and my brothers, following my mother's move, the four of us went to a beautiful concert and afterward we cried together under the starry sky.

With grief *and* with happiness.

With pain *and* love.

I'm still crying.

In spite of everything and thanks to everything.

CONCLUSION

It's now up to me to keep remembering my mother, to keep giving her an active place in my life. I want to affirm her impact in who I am and everything I do. I could have done without the dementia, but she's not her illness. She's a human being. She's my mom.

I'll never forget that time when we lay in the dunes, enjoying the sun together, and how happy she was by the sea. The sound of her whistling, which my brothers and I would recognize from miles away as the signal to go home. I won't forget her winning every trivia quiz, finding the empty licorice jar beside her chair in the morning, and her inability to walk past a bookshop without browsing for hours. And how could I forget that she gave me a sticker book after I got my finger caught in the door, the sight of her in the front seat of the car, her smell, her laugh, and her fierce dark gaze.

I can still see myself lying on the purple floral bedspread while my mom is folding the laundry. I'm so young and she's so grown up. Everything has been ironed, even the wash-cloths. The scent of detergent lingers in the room as I watch her. I'm just lying there. We're together, my mother and me.

My mom.

Nothing much was said during those moments.

Even back then that was more than enough.

You're still in the spring of life
all love and smiles and sun
still free from fear and pain
and sorrows yet unknown

A life still full of joy and light
birdsong in the month of May
ladybugs and butterflies
vibrant as a brand-new day

But spring, alas, it cannot last,
and change is on the wind
May gives way to autumn rain,
this reveling will end

Unless you always treasure
and forever keep alive
the memories of these golden days
this sun-filled time of life

My mother's entry in my friendship book
(1988–89)

ACKNOWLEDGMENTS

I want to start by thanking you. Thank you for your trust and your time. I don't know you personally, but the dementia of our loved ones has enabled us to cross paths. I hope that you've found some glimmers of hope in my words, and that in turn you will share the rays of light that you discover with the people you encounter along the way. If we all do that, the story of dementia will become more transparent and more complete. That's crucial. It may provide comfort and encouragement to others. By joining forces, we can create an entire galaxy of light—visible from far and wide to all those who come looking for it.

I owe a debt of gratitude to all those in my immediate surroundings who have or had a loved one with dementia and who shared their vulnerable stories and feelings with me: Our shared experiences have touched, inspired, and spurred me on during the writing of this book.

I want to thank my parents, who've always encouraged me to search for meaning. Thanks, Dad, for showing what love for better or worse really means. Thank you, Mom, for who you are, for the lessons you keep teaching me. And just in case you haven't been able to read it between the lines: I'm immensely grateful to my brothers. They mean the world to me. We're incredibly lucky to be part of this family, but we also make a big effort to spend time together and to keep loving and supporting one another—not just when it's all fun and games, but also and especially when things aren't going so well. Of course, I'm also grateful to my two sons. They're my bedrock, and they pull me back into real life whenever I disappear behind my laptop into a world of words and stories. I'm grateful to my partner and my friends—knowing that they've chosen to be part of my life is true happiness.

My family would like to thank the nursing home and in particular the caregivers on my mother's ward. Their professional assistance and the love and tenderness with which they surround her are priceless. Words can't express how important and valuable their work is. Our thanks also to the social worker for the comfort and encouragement she offers my father and for the wisdom and insights she was prepared to share with me.

Thank you, Hedi, my Dutch editor, for providing a critical voice and gentle motivation. You know what it means to find dementia on your path, as does Annelinde, the Dutch art director who gave this book its original design. Your personal connection to this topic is palpable on every page.

Thank you, Martine, for your faith in this book and in my story. Thank you, Maaike, for the publicity. I want to thank Laurie at Kosmos, while Julia at Shared Stories also deserves a heartfelt thank you.

FURTHER READING

First and foremost, I've drawn on the people around me, who shared their experiences, insights, and emotions about dealing with dementia—these unwritten, real-life stories have been woven into *When a Loved One Has Dementia*.

The epigraph on page iii is from *Iedereen was er. Meer verhalen over de eekhoorn en de andere dieren* ("Everybody Was There: More Stories about the Squirrel and the Other Creatures") by Toon Tellegen. The advice on page 134 was adapted, with permission, from a text by Saskia Vullers from leafritueelbegeleiding.nl.

The books that I've quoted from the most, because they were invaluable in giving me a better understanding of both my mother's diagnosis and the actual illness, are as follows.

Buijssen, Huub. *The Simplicity of Dementia: A Guide for Family and Carers* (London: Jessica Kingsley Publishers, 2005).

Gerrard, Nicci. *The Last Ocean: What Dementia Teaches Us About Love* (New York: Penguin, 2020).

Hall, Jan. *Dementia Essentials: How to Guide a Loved One Through Alzheimer's or Dementia and Provide the Best Care* (New York: Vermilion, 2013; reprinted 2021).

ADDITIONAL BOOKS

Andrews, June. *Dementia, The One-Stop Guide* (New York: Profile Books, 2015).

Atkins, Simon. *Dementia for Dummies* (New York: Wiley, 2015).

Buijssen, Huub. *Het hart wordt niet dement* ("The Heart of Dementia"; Tilburg, NL: Buijssen Training en Educatie, 2019).

Devine, Megan. *It's OK That You're Not OK: Meeting Grief and Loss in a Culture that Doesn't Understand* (Louisville, CO: Sounds True, 2017).

Draaisma, Douwe. *The Nostalgia Factory: Memory, Time and Ageing* (New Haven, CT: Yale University Press, 2013).

Eger, Dr. Edith Eva. *The Choice: Embrace the Possible* (New York: Scribner, 2017).

Genova, Lisa. *Still Alice* (New York: Pocket Books, 2009; adapted as a film in 2014).

Kübler-Ross, Elisabeth, and David Kessler. *On Grief and Grieving* (New York: Simon & Schuster, 2005).

Lesser, Elizabeth. *Broken Open* (New York: Villard, 2004).

Stolp, Hans. *De verborgen zin van dementie* ("The Hidden Meaning of Dementia"; Utrecht, NL: AnkhHermes, 2015).

Strayed, Cheryl. *Tiny Beautiful Things* (New York: Vintage, 2012).

Swaab, Dick. *We Are Our Brains: From the Womb to Alzheimer's* (New York: Penguin, 2015).

Swinton, John. *Dementia: Living in the Memories of God* (Grand Rapids, MI: Eerdmans, 2012).

RESOURCES

Alzheimer's Association: alz.org

Alzheimers.gov: alzheimers.gov

Alzheimer's Foundation of America: alzfdn.org

Family Caregiver Alliance: caregiver.org

National Aphasia Association: aphasia.org

National Institute on Aging: nia.nih.gov

American Brain Foundation: americanbrainfoundation.org

ABOUT THE AUTHOR AND TRANSLATOR

EVELINE HELMINK is a licensed coach practitioner, working one-on-one with clients on themes such as grief, change, and acceptance. She is also a journalist, magazine editor, and the author of *The Handbook for Bad Days*. She works as an editor in chief at the international media brand Happinez, which shares insights and inspiration for personal growth and a meaningful life. Her mother lives with dementia. She lives in Amsterdam, the Netherlands.

⊙ eveline.helmink

LAURA VROOMEN has been a translator from Dutch for twenty years. She translates fiction and nonfiction and has tackled a diverse range of topics, including mindfulness, food, and the environment. She lives in Glasgow, Scotland.